the *Posh Girl's* GUIDE TO PLAY

fantasy, role play,
and sensual bondage

ALEXIS LASS

SEAL PRESS

THE POSH GIRL'S GUIDE TO PLAY
Fantasy, Role Play, and Sensual Bondage

Seal Press
Copyright © 2013 Alexis Lass
Published by
Seal Press
A Member of the Perseus Books Group
1700 Fourth Street
Berkeley, California
www.sealpress.com

Library of Congress Cataloging-in-Publication Data

Lass, Alexis.
Posh girl's guide to play : fantasy, role play, and sensual bondage / by Alexis Lass.
pages cm
ISBN 978-1-58005-525-3
1. Women—Sexual behavior. I. Title.
HQ29.L37 2013
306.7082—dc23
2013016151

9 8 7 6 5 4 3 2 1

Cover and interior design by Domini Dragoone
Printed in the United States of America
Distributed by Publishers Group West

AUTHOR'S NOTE

THROUGHOUT THIS GUIDE, UPON REQUEST, OR as I have seen fit, I refer to story participants, friends, and sources by a single initial, arbitrarily chosen. In a few instances, I have changed identifying characteristics—gender, nationality, physical appearance, locale, and other descriptive details—to preserve the anonymity of those same individuals. From some, I asked permission to use their words. Others are quoted in paraphrase and/or portrayed from my recollections.

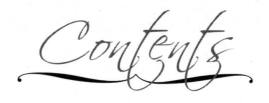

Contents

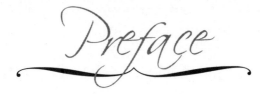

Preface

"*Women . . . too have their pornography: Harlequin romances, novels of 'sweet savagery,' bodice-rippers.*"
—THE NEW YORK TIMES, DECEMBER 1980

Some thirty-odd years after these words were written, *Fifty Shades of Grey* author E. L. James has given us far more than ripped bodices. She has ripped the plain brown wrapper off erotic fem lit and normalized the conversation around dominance and submission for women everywhere.

And I should know. Raised on New York City's Upper East Side and schooled at Spence (all girls) and the Kent School (boarding school, the horsey set, in Connecticut), I grew up in a cloistered, conservative world of privilege and politesse. But in my early twenties, I was ready for adventure and took that desire further than anyone (and that includes me) might have guessed: I walked into an S&M dungeon and began my training as a professional dominatrix. After five years as Domme Dietrich, I launched my own fetish film company, Firefive Productions.

And then, at long last, I myself—skittish about my own sexual vulner-ability despite my pro domme experience—learned to submit, at the talented hands of a certain Mr. H, whom you'll meet soon enough.

But we've time for all that. First it must be said that as earthshak-ing an influence as E. L. James has had of late, she didn't invent the (spiked) wheel. Dominance and submission in social and sexual practice is age-old, dating to early human history, when the hunter (male)/gath-erer (female) roles were defined by the life-and-death realities of sur-vival. Dare we say, when men were men? Conking the wildebeest over the head before dragging his chosen off to the cave—"Me Tarzan, you Jane." And from there it's not a far stretch to that iconic scene in which Rhett Butler forcefully sweeps Scarlett O'Hara off her feet and hauls her up that decadent staircase to warm the marital bed (recall, as well, her morning-after expression of pure "guilty pleasure"). Then there are the trailblazing *Story of O*, the off-Broadway sensation *Venus in Fur*, the films *9½ Weeks* and *Secretary*, and, from the daddy of them all, the Marquis de Sade, his masterwork of S&M, *Justine*.

That is to say, if you're curious about the world of dominance and submission, you are in fine cultural company. But fiction hasn't really told us *how to live* in that world—how to enter it safely, how to relish its powers, and how to cast it off like a party dress when (and if) you're done. Similarly, even the most compelling literary or cinematic heroine isn't the same as a trusted source. Reading is not doing. Reel life isn't real life.

Enter *The Posh Girl's Guide to Play*. You might think of this hand-book as the posh girl's, the thoroughbred woman's, home companion to S&M: a glittering passage into your own erotically playful world—a real world wherein you may indulge the fantasies you've been living vicari-ously through the tease of tantalizing accounts featuring fictional char-acters. And I invite you to think of me as your posh play Virgil—from Spence to spanking, debutantes to dungeons, I've covered this territory, and I can tell you that the journey will be delicious.

To help me serve your kinky best interests, I've begged the help of a special man of mine: Mr. H. Anonymous for the purposes of this book, to guard his "vanilla" life, Mr. H is a tall, dark, and handsome male dom who also has run a successful blog on S&M role play. He was my own personal Virgil, and I thank him for teaching me how to submit and how to love it.

In an effort to pay his wickedness forward, I promise, through this book and with his generous help, to teach you how to draw out the Mr. H (or, if you prefer, the Christian Grey) in your very own man.

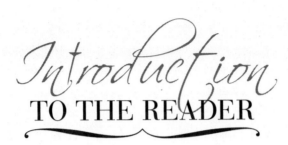

Introduction
TO THE READER

My childhood and adolescence—which involved more inter-actions with horses than with members of the opposite sex—tracked an unlikely prelude to the aforementioned mores-breaking, renegade decision I made in my early twenties: to apply for a dom-inatrix job at a New York City dungeon. Whoaaa! Back up! Okay: I had just returned from a summer session at the University of Bologna and travels through Italy with a girlfriend who'd been a classmate at Bard College. We'd worn Venetian masks for fun at Vivaldi concerts and giggled while everyone stared at us, smoked European cigarettes atop elaborate sculptured fountains. Then off we'd gone to Paris for dancing in Left Bank nightclubs and to Switzerland for gorging on chocolate, on our parents' dime.

Arriving home from my year of lush and louche fun, I enrolled in acting school, wanting to prove to my parents I could make it on my own as an artist. Like every actress, I needed an evening job so I could run off to auditions during the day. Instead of the cliché waitress gig, I decided to try something offbeat and darkly glamorous, a job a boy-friend suggested I would be "great at."

Walking into that New York City dungeon, with rooms elaborately decked out to look like replicas of the Marquis de Sade's castle chambers . . . hmmmm. I felt as if I were on a noir film set—a dream come true for an aspirational filmmaker and artist. It intrigued me from the get-go. During my interview with the dungeon master, I saw beautiful young women walking men on dog leashes, a man prancing around in full drag (in Agent Provocateur lingerie, no less), and all sorts of wild, scary, and delectable new toys in this castle of posh doom and decadence. Terrified but excited, I was thrown to the lions—no apprenticeship. In my first session with a sub male, I had no idea what I was doing, what was expected, but was told he desperately wanted to be tied to a glistening black cross and whipped. Wearing Mother's Chanel leather suit (gainfully repurposed, as it were), whip in hand, I was off and whipping my submissive captive, who revealed after the session that he was a well-known Broadway playwright (shhhh!). Thus began my five-year career as a dominatrix (or pro domme, as they say in the trade), played out in the dungeon and subsequently on film sets of videos I produced for my next venture, an online fetish-film site.

A multimillionaire, to-the-British-manor-born male sub fronted me a hefty sum to launch Firefive Productions, our co-owned fetish film company in Manhattan. The movies we made explored every imaginable role-play scenario to satisfy customer demand. I heartily ditched acting to create and direct my own David Lynch–y, high-end, li'l kinky films. Immersed in S&M, and playing the embedded correspondent on the front lines, I undertook a talent-scouting mission and a hunt for the true grit.

I started attending all the secret fetish parties in New York's S&M underworld and was surprised to find myself in the company of so many of the city's Masters of the Universe. These were powerful, domineering men by day, being dominated by, or sometimes dominating (a man may be a submissive, a dom, or a switch), mostly beautiful young women wearing the sort of $2,000 shiny black latex catsuits that might be seen on Lady Gaga. The women's party wardrobes were

Gucci dresses paired with Alexander McQueen thigh-high black stiletto boots, accessorized by elegant long leather gloves, custom-made Australian whips, and kinky toys tucked into their French handbags. The women were more Hollywood silver screen-ready than a roomful of actual Hollywood starlets. The scene was über-glamorous and decadent and, for me, more *Eyes Wide Shocked* than *Eyes Wide Shut*. I attended secret parties where gorgeous women and Wall Street's financial powerhouses engaged in all sorts of kinky role play. In one room, I'd see a pretty girl tied with rope, dangling from a suspension device, looking like an airborne nude ballerina as she was defiled by her handsome male dom, who paddled and sexually manhandled her; in the next, I'd see Catwomen whipping a naked couple tied to each other and simultaneously moaning in endorphin-releasing delight; and much more startling kink. All done in "public" while players and masked gawkers (some of them mega A-list celebrities in hiding—whose names I shall leave out—and many more middle-income school teachers, lawyers, and other professionals) sipped expensive Champagnes and wines. The rule scrupulously observed at a clandestine S&M party, as in a dungeon, is that no real names are used, whether you're a car mechanic or a supermodel. You're simply Mistress von Kink or Sub Ophelia, Master Versailles or Sub John—no true identities and no telling tales in the daytime, "vanilla" world. This is how everyone—average Joe or celeb, struggling actress or Fortune 500 rich guy—can safely let his or her wildest kinky desires play out without having to worry about ending up on Page Six the next morning.

And onward, to the guide. But first off, the author takes a question:

Q. Who the hell do you think you are, writing about the subject of dominant and submissive role play (DSRP)?

A. Did Dr. Kinsey hand me a PhD in human sexuality? Am I licensed to teach sex ed to the country's randy high school freshmen? Nope and nope. Not certified, not interested. What I am is an ex–pro dominatrix who worked in New York City's most sensational dungeon and ran my own online fetish film business; a sensual role-play advocate and practitioner who's played on both sides of the paddle; and an unabashed sensualist who's learned a thing or two in the field and between the sheets. Also, I have a frisky imagination that leans toward the artistic, and I keep good company. (You'll meet the guy-guide, my BF, and peerless accomplice, Mr. H.)

And, next, a quick note about the guide's structure and some thoughts on the ways you may choose to read it. Each chapter is a mix of show 'n' tell—primer text on the various elements of DSRP, advice and counsel, and storytelling—ending with suggested warm-up exercises. There's a progressive intensity to play action. You might zip through to the endgame (beware chapter 12, which is all about "Taboos"!) and then revisit each chapter to work through the exercises. Or, you may prefer to take things step by step through the graduated levels, putting new concepts into practice as you go. Some eager readers may be tempted to plunge directly into the guide's "red-light district of super-kink," but I caution against it because it's the finale for good reason. As a greenhorn, do you really want to tackle bronco busting before you master a slow canter around the ring? Throughout the book, Mr. H and I, incorporating much valuable feedback from women who play, offer wise cautionary words on the choosing of play partners, the setting of limits, trusting your gut, and, well, keeping things playful. In the words of my good guy friend N, "If you don't listen to your gut, you're gonna regret it. Your brain's not that bright and your heart is an idiot." These better-safe-than-sorry refrains, tailored to each graduated step of the DSRP caper, are critical body-, soul-, and face-saving prelims to satisfying adventure.

And one last thing before I get on with it. For me, BDSM belongs to the realm of art, whereas so much of our lives is lived on the planes of animal and vegetable. Eating. Drinking. Peeing. Sleeping. Even, for most people, most of the time, fucking—which in a wilting relationship becomes just another rudimentary, physical action, like scratching an itch. That said, I qualify: I'm chill with the B (bondage) and D (dominance/discipline) of that scary acronym BDSM, but I'm no masochist and my lover(s) is (are) no sadist(s). S&M is an archaic and rusty term that does *not* represent all or most popular dominant and submissive role play. Which isn't to say we're not gonna get kinky, not gonna get crazy—we are! But nothing plucked from the psycho torture toy chest. This guide is intended for the adventurous, whole, and healthy woman who prefers life with a twist . . . stirred not shaken, *s'il vous plaît*.

Now, playing outside the dungeon, in private and with a trusted partner, you will not have the worry of being "outed." You may, however, have other concerns or misgivings, and you may be wondering if DSRP is for you. Herewith, I try to address all these issues.

REASONS TO EXPLORE DSRP (BDSM):
Do any of these describe you?

1. I want to try something new, explore, and get to know myself.
2. I have experience with BDSM but I'd like to discover and learn more.
3. I was really getting into BDSM, and then I had a bad experience. I wish I knew what went wrong so I could continue to enjoy the practice.
4. I am BDSM-curious and entertain related fantasies.
5. I thought *Fifty Shades of Grey* was hot and romantic and I want to try BDSM play.
6. My lover and I are fighting too much, and it's taxing our relationship.
7. I would love to tone down the stress in my life.
8. I am a dominant female and I'm wondering how it would feel to be relieved of control and play a submissive role in a "tryout" play experience.
9. I have taken yoga classes and they satisfy me in a way that typical gym exercise classes do not.
10. My relationship has gone sexually stale and/or my lover has a small dinky and I can't deal.

If your answer is yes to any of these statements, then this guide is for you.

COMMON FEARS:

Do any of these describe you?

1. I'm scared my lover will not share, or will be turned off by, my desire to try BDSM.

2. I'm afraid that if I try BDSM play with my lover and it's an embarrassing experience, I will wreck the relationship and regret my advances.

3. I'm nervous and a little embarrassed about even mentioning my BDSM fantasies and desires to explore this play.

4. I always thought that S&M and BDSM were for extreme, weird people, and that they were kinda sick.

5. I'm a feminist and I think being submissive to a man, even in a temporary play experience, is antifeminist and unhealthy for women.

6. I'm afraid I might get physically or emotionally hurt during BDSM play.

7. I think my religion would regard BDSM play as impure, sinful, and unnatural.

8. I'm feeling uncomfortable with some of the accessories and practices of BDSM play: the kinky costumes, the use of crops, paddles, handcuffs, and other kinky toys, and addressing my lover as "Master."

9. I worry that practicing BDSM play will label me a fetishist. I'm even second-guessing myself, wondering whether just being attracted to it means I have a fetish.

10. I secretly think my S&M fantasy or fantasies are crazy-abnormal-f'd up . . . eek!

The most straightforward response to all the above concerns and hypothetical fears is "Don't worry." These are common misgivings, reflecting the prevalent myths advanced by online and pop media, talk shows, and various publications to stigmatize what can be a wholesome, romantic, and invigorating sexual practice. For the Posh Girl's response to *all that*, read on! All concerns itemized above will be more fully addressed within the guide.

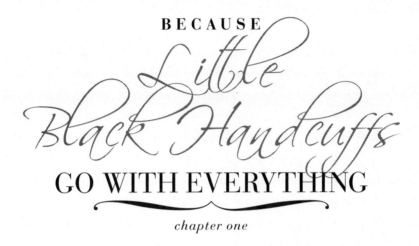

GO WITH EVERYTHING

chapter one

Here's to you, feminista moms everywhere. Thanks for
everything, really. R-e-a-l-l-y. You marched, you rallied,
you sacked the laddie citadels for us, torched those bras
for us. And I grab the mic on behalf of all your daughters
to roar: Those bras did not die in vain, dammit! We work,
we earn, we compete, we kick ass! And now we'd
like to, y'know, play for a bit . . .

Yes, Play is the name of this game. And BDSM is the name of the
playground. But not *r-e-a-l-l-y*. Keeping things Posh, in these pages
we'll frolic on the sensually pleasurable fringes and avoid the tortur-
ous shoals of "play," which is dungeon-speak for the sometimes brutal
activities that go on in a pay-to-play dungeon. Our play will be seriously
fun, sexually charged role play. *But.* We're meant for the stage, *grande
dames*, not the meat locker. In this world, you'll get to *act*. To star in your
own production. You'll be writer, director, set designer, and wardrobe

and props mistress, pardon the pun. In creating roles for yourself and a trusted partner, you will improvise dialogue and steer the scene in ways that suit you. It's not just "lick faster, lick slower"—you'll use *creativity* to excite the other person.

Starring in the role of Subordinated Damsel, you'll find that the sexy "You Tarzan, me Jane" playlet can pay surprising, climactic (!) rewards: thrills 'n' chills that shake up Real Life with an exhilarating bust-out from the jail of dreary routine.

If you're with me—and why else open *this* book—you've likely read, or read about, or read your BFF's dog-eared pages of *that* book. (Okay, let's just get it out there: We're talking *Fifty Shades of Grey*, the BDSM-flavored niche erotica that refused to stay niched, hereinafter simply "that book.") And it spoke to you. And you're curious. Tempted. Daring enough to explore the tantalizing possibilities of what only yesterday seemed forbidden territory.

Hard to imagine now, but sex itself, or at least sex as recreation, was a closeted idea back in the day. As director David Cronenberg exulted, in words I recall reading—and loving—around the time his movie *Crash* was released (and here, I paraphrase, because I can't source the quote): At the time contraception came in, sex . . . left biology and entered the realm of culture. It was about what we chose for pleasure rather than what we did for reproduction.

Lucky, lucky us.

I LEAD OFF WITH A QUESTION: Have you ever fantasized about dominant and submissive sensual role play?

Ha! I'm hearing a chorus of *duhs*, but it is a central question, because sensual role play derives from, and builds on, a rich fantasy life. Meaning the stuff of dreams, not nightmares. No dank dungeons, lethal whips, clunky chains, cheesy, fussy handcuffs, Spike's spiked collar and leash, hefty paddles, electrodes, sharp metal nipple clamps, masters beating slaves into submission. Eek! No, no, no, and *no*! Indulging in DSRP should be a delight, not a torture. It shouldn't leave you nursing wounds to your body or your pride, and how could it, Madame Director? You're pulling the strings (offscreen) so that your partner may take charge (on the set). Fliply (and for your eyes only!), you might think of it this way: You, Pavlov, zap the testosterone. He, well-conditioned, eager-to-please lab pup, performs.

We're going to jazz up the quaint notion of guy on top (as nature intended? Ha! We're selfishly exercising free will here.). We're going to facilitate his dominating a compliant you by means of your own private fantasy scenarios. Boudoir soft-tools may be your stockings or panties, his neckties, and other household props serving as bondage toys. An open palm works just fine in the delivery of old-fashioned hand-spanking punishment. Sound more inviting, a more thinkable arsenal, than hard-core artillery? I concur. Kink toys off the triple-X shelf might be a fun, cool buy and may enhance play for some, and if you're into that stuff, go girl! But *please* don't consider S&M merchandise as the only starter kit to sexual kink play. That's the BS too many kink guidebooks slap you into thinking. *Sighs.* The exercise of DSRP does not require you to Google a glossary of S&M terms or buy a toy chest of tools. The way this girl likes it is *au naturel*, hard and hot but nothing that makes me wrinkle my nose (butt plugs? *ewwww*) or call for the EMTs (metal-tipped floggers). No.

PLEASE ALLOW ME, IN THESE EARLY chapters, to introduce some comfortable, real-deal concepts underlying the sensual and naturally delicious world of kinky DSRP. It can be so-o-o-o good! You may find, as I have, that role play relieves the pent-up, demoralizing, even crippling frustration, stress, and anxieties experienced by modern women—pretty much all of us, from working girls to stay-at-home moms. I find it tantamount to the great yoga workout that offers physical and mental release through unorthodox body stretches, under the direction of an enthusiastic and skillful instructor/master. DSRP should be practiced as a wholesome, exciting exercise that can enliven your relationships by allowing you to dig deep into you, to discover what you may have despaired of ever having: strengthened confidence in relations with your lover, heightened courage, better emotional balance, and new and useful perspectives on what makes *you* tick, with a bonus payoff in stress management. And, oh yeah, lots of fun!

For a vividly apt, cinematic metaphor, I offer the blood-pumping, edge-of-your-seat thrills of a horror movie. None of us voyeurs really wants to be killed by the fat guy with the chainsaw chasing us through a cornfield. But we like *feeling* as if we *might* be killed in the cornfield by the fat guy with the chainsaw. For the moment, as we shudder in the role of chasee, the sensation of fright is real, but we always know we are in a movie seat and that we will leave the theater unharmed. Visualization, a powerful tool in DSRP, can conjure the same state of arousal: electrifying and thrilling yet *safe*—sweet! And I trust you'll come up with something hotter than a lumbering maniac with dishonorable intentions.

WHAT IF YOU'RE LIKE ME, INITIALLY nervous about unleashing the "dirty" desires that "proper girls" don't talk about, let alone—*horreurs!*—indulge?

Think back to the evening of 12/21/12.

The Mayan apocalypse hoopla was a hot excuse for women to say "screw it" and toss their sexual inhibitions out like last year's expensive panties. The tabloids reported polls showing that a lot of "nice girls" had decided to get reckless and "kinky." They gleefully told researchers, in so many words, "We're throwing out the missionary with the bath water, going for the 'kinky' for our last bacchanal poke before being blitz-o'ed." Sounds like a handy excuse to kick out, to me, but good for them! (And my bet is that not one of those breaker-outers who acted on their fantasies suffered morning-after regrets—*they were ready!*)

The message here is that whatever may be on your D-day list of things to hit—so satisfying to tick off line items, even on the grocery list, no?—get moving! Not every calendar date presents an opportunity for D-day girls-gone-rogue, but why should any of us need an apocalypse-grade excuse to indulge our sexual desires? Let that pent-up shit go, for heaven's sake—for your *own* sake! Relax and take advantage of that feminista mom's hard-won freedom to enjoy yourself.

Recall to mind, here, one of those dithering flip-flop moments like, "Should I—I can't—but oh hell, screw it—I *will* splurge on that luxurious vacation!" You book the tickets and you do fly the hell out of your ho-hum comfort zone to the delightful otherness of a holiday. Good show! What's a couple of weeks living on Frappuccinos compared to the infinite possibilities of adventure? I'll tell you: You won't remember the former, and the latter may change your life. That's what. And what's more, novelty and unpredictability fire up the brain's rewards center like little miracles—it's all about the dopamine, a.k.a. our "pleasure chemical," as DSRP practitioners well know.

Yep. I've found that adventurous DSRP ignites the pleasure zones in much the same way as the fun and release of a vacation. Even the indulging of an extravagant D-day-list fantasy can be that blissful vacation—an escape, a kiss-off to monotony, a sexual reset of the old in-and-out stagnation.

An aside, drawn from my own fantasy repertoire, if I may. Two of my favorite English words are *lagoon* and *taboo*. Both are loaded with sexy suggestion. Both are double-*O* words that command the lips to pucker up. Speak them slowly, softly to yourself, eyes closed. Conjure the sensual pleasure of a lush, secluded paradise and the tingle of a romp in forbidden territory. Are we there yet? Brava! You're in Posh Girl Playland.

This, then, is how transporting sensual role play can feel when done surefootedly, with foreknowledge of the practice, some polished skills, and the natural-ability trump card that biology deals most females (dare we call it "wiles"?). The upshot is that role play draws on your imagination rather than your bank account—the guiltless getaway.

One of the goals of this book is to usher you to a state of confidence in which you can simply close your eyes, summon your full store of sensory memories, and let the play flow through—technique straight out of the *Kama Sutra* vault.

IN THE SUCCEEDING CHAPTERS OF THIS guide, sensual role play is wrapped up as just such a glam vacation package, delivered with a gift basket of practical suggestions, skills, and exercises—field-tested tools of the trade that will help you start your spicy vacation off on the right foot. I will explain

- how to prepare yourself for this new world of play, emotionally and physically;
- how to find or create your own approach to and style of role play, with or without DIY and over-the-kinkshop-counter toys;
- how to plan for a safe, smooth ride: an unclunky, unclumsy play experience sans embarrassment (promise!); and
- how to get things rolling, detailing the many ways and means of telling your lover you wish to play—seamlessly, with assurance, without scarlet cheeks.

TAKING THAT FIRST STEP, I MUST admit, was the hardest bit for me, just nail-biting hell. Even now, after *that book* has put role play into universal play, it takes some guts to "confess" to partners that, for instance, one likes being spanked. (No! I wasn't abused as a child, and No! I definitely, decidedly do not see you as *daddy*, and Yes! all this fun-and-games stuff ends at the breakfast table.) But, as I learned through trial and many errors (some quite comical, as you'll see), there are ways of breaking the ice so as not to embarrass yourself or your partner into capillary-pounding awkwardness. For the ultra-skittish, the easiest way out may be this: shoot your man a quick text to visit the Posh Girl's Guide website: littleblackhandcuffs.com. In a section for guys, my partner Mr. H guides the newbies through a BDSM crash course. Simple. Bam! Done. In the following chapters, I will share all of it, learned firsthand and also through story-trading. No worries: I contend that if this ultra-squeamish, conservatively reared girl (see preface) can master it, you can, too. Yes, yes, *that book* helped beyond measure in bringing BDSM out of the psycho-girl snakepit.

Busting down the door to mainstream acceptance. Helping to demystify DSRP, certainly. But now we need to delve into how exactly one is to execute all this new titillating role play.

My male partner and guide contributor, the accomplished Mr. H, and I recently have fortified his manly stylized blog, HIsfortheHunter.blogspot.com, launched in 2001, with instructions for the guys—partners and husbands—who seemed suddenly full of questions and eager to learn about sensual role play. No mystery here: It was about the same time *that book* exploded and became the talk of the town, hell, the Western world. Mr. H and I saw it as a great development, as the queries from men centered on how to give *you* what you want. The blog material—written by Mr. H in a coolly clinical, "What's up, man, here's what chicks like and don't like in role play" fashion, dude to dude—was a tremendous contribution to this guide. All you squeamish girls (remember, that includes *moi*) need do is text your guy the link and let him take it from there. It's a much slicker idea than leaving a cliché gray tie on his side of the bed, as I've heard some desperate housewives have tried. That's cute but doesn't do it. So your man picks up the damn tie, maybe gets the reference, maybe channels the (im)proper message. Then what? Imagine what a stand-up comedian could do with this material: "Oh shit, oh lord, I'm in trouble! Whaddaya want here, anyway? I make a noose and what? Hang myself? Hang the babysitter? Fer f's sake, woman, can't ya just *tell* me what the hell it is you want?" Poor chap hasn't a clue. And how could he? It's your fantasy, your show, and here he is, standing like a dope without a playbill.

That opening gambit is perhaps the trickiest hurdle, but it doesn't have to go down like this. Once you hack into chapter 2 ("Breaking the Ice"), a dialogue-based tutorial on "spilling," once you buck up and muster your resources, it's olly olly oxen free . . . *CHARGE!* You'll be proud of yourself for being bold, and, setting your sights on the grand prize, you'll be ready to start putting the play into play.

MEANWHILE, SOME CLARIFYING WORDS.

What dominant/submissive role play (DSRP) is *not* (in *my* book and in *this* book):

I'm not going to give you a hair-raising fright history of BDSM or S&M. (Eye roll permitted.) Yes, we all know about the torture chambers and the wicked exploits of the Marquis de Sade, who, charmingly, lent his surname to a textbook term in our kink vocabulary. Much more in the spirit of our inquiry here are the bawdy escapades of fifties glam naughty girl Bettie Paige and the riveting carryings-on of the title role character in the BDSM-themed movie *Secretary*, both of which are more useful models for couples who wish to participate in non-extremist DSRP. The key word is *play*, defined by me as a rousingly fun sexual sideline one engages in from time to time without bolting off the cliff into obsession territory. (Whereupon the word becomes *fetish*.)

Throughout the guide, I reference the self-imposed boundaries and limits I've set and recommend to all for a safe, sane, and enjoyable venture into this bountiful, beguiling garden. It beckons with oh-so-pretty roses and some mighty ugly thorns.

What DSRP *is*: DSRP is a variant of sexual practice in which one partner physically and mentally dominates the other, by mutual consent and in a mutual desire to please, the rewards being a robust boost to emotional and relationship balance, relaxation, self-awareness and, of course, a heightening of the sexual experience (from my custom-tailored dictionary).

Balance: You will find that, in fact, the submissive in healthy role play controls the dominant by setting—and enforcing—limits for her dominant. Funny, in submitting to your dominant lover, yours is the stronger role. A courageous and open one. Sexual submission is openness. Openness is not weakness. Submission is not weakness. In turn, the nominal dominant partner effectively becomes the submissive in that he is consumed and dominated by his submissive's desires. In trying to sort things out, toy with the notion of "illusion," that is, a fantasy or idea that results in a mistaken perception of reality, and you'll find that your reality is mutable. Who's really in control? The answer is you both are.

Relaxation: Yes, yes, this play is intense and the stakes high-tension titillation. So how can it be relaxing? Well, most women experience sensual role play as so high-powered that after the initial explosion, there's a settling down. Recent activities play out deep in the mind, and the body relaxes, does a metaphorical exhale. (Though I hasten to add that the aftershocks are glorious and can keep you smiling for days!) I think you'll find that role play is a surefire trigger to this heightened intensity, well beyond the levels experienced during routine sexual activity. A good analogy may be the letting-go exhilaration one feels after a free fall from the pinnacle of a roller coaster. As with a meditation session, it's eyes closed, brain off, submitting to the unknown, beyond the clutter of your normal racing brain. You'll find the sensations similar to those you feel in submitting to the ministrations of a talented masseuse. As you lie there, facedown, naked and vulnerable, surrendering, submitting, you relax into the otherworldly pleasure of what's technically domination by another.

Self-awareness: We are creatures of oxygen and sex: We breathe, we mate; it's how we survive. It's when we dance away from the basics and indulge our sexual fancies that we plug into our motherboard psychology and begin to learn what makes us tick. Why do we prefer this or that particular sexual fantasy? Must we explain or defend? In the wise words of sex therapist and neuroscientist Nan Wise, who studies the brain at orgasm, "Nature loves diversity and society abhors it. There are many, many ways that people are wired for pleasure. We all have unique erotic fingerprints."[1]

Heightened sexual experience: Though sexuality generally remains a private part of our lives, engaging in sex is one of the few activities that encourages us to get primal, to act with the joyous natural abandon of our unselfconscious mammal cousins.

Let's just face it, sex is a bit aggro.

If you follow the guide, chew on the commentary, make the stories your own, and put into practice the knowledge you need to customize your role, keeping things safe and consensual, you're on your way to sexual nirvana. Nature's got the formula, you have the control, and I hope to hand you the tools to make your man play hard (or soft). Big new orgasms mean happy couples. Cheers!

Exercises

1. Start with a simple Google search. Try "free erotic sub girl stories." Or try "BDSM sub girl fiction"—there's a ton of hot S&M erotic fiction online. Alternatively, start with a book—one of the classics, such as *Story of O* by Pauline Réage, *L'Image* by Catherine Robbe-Grillet, The Sleeping Beauty Trilogy by Anne Rice writing as A. N. Roquelaure (great erotic book), or, of *coooourse*, the blockbuster hit-o-rama *Fifty Shades of Grey*. Look at both published books and the amateur blogs, as most online stories have more hardcore, gritty action. Get a wide-ranging sense of everything under the whip. Then ask yourself:

   What scenes or specific actions did I like the most?
   What scenes or specific actions creeped me out or didn't turn me on?

   Next, make a list of all the role-play actions you did not like and think you would not enjoy (e.g., the use of sex toys or pain toys, having my legs tied to bed posts, having a gag in my mouth, being called a "___," being paddled). Make a note of why these scenes didn't appeal to you (e.g., these parts were too rough for me, these words and actions were cheesy, etc.) Or at least make a mental list and remember it.

2. Write out your own erotic submissive-girl role-play fantasy story or scene. Add as much information as possible, down to a description of your fantasy dominant lover, what you are wearing to turn him on, the

location of the encounter, and every action in detail. You can certainly steal scenes from the erotic stories you've read and customize them. Make them your own. Give yourself fifteen minutes to write this fantasy story or scene. A professor friend at New York University told me she gives her students fifteen minutes to write on a subject. She finds that her students don't overthink their pieces or humor their inhibitions when constrained to a short time frame, and that some students write their best stuff under these conditions. You can revisit the story, revising and expanding, as new thoughts occur.

When you're done, perhaps even submit your scene to a blog or start your own anonymous erotic story blog.[2]

I WILL START YOU OFF WITH an erotic story you might fancy and that might help stir your budding erotic imagination.

It's a story I'll teasingly call "The Story of J." With reality always being stranger than fiction, and this story being 100 percent reality, the tale hangs on the tongue like a slice of sizzling, rare meat—raw, enticing, and tender to the bite. It is, if anything, the ultimate example of a thrill ride—a true crime experience that, while real, was anything but honest. It's a tale of how the burning dark corners of the imagination can spice up one's sex life in ways one might never suspect. I will use fake names to protect the guilty and the sinless. I'll add in some atmosphere but I'll keep all the facts exactly as they happened. Be forewarned and fore-delighted.

This happened to my mother's first cousin, a woman I'll call J, in the 1970s, when conspiracy theories about the government were at their peak and New York City was at its most lawless, with heart-stopping dangers (and thrills) lurking in every neighborhood. J was not your blueprint blue-eyed, blond Midwestern beauty queen, though she was a Hoosier, and beautiful (green eyes, strawberry-blond hair, flawless skin, elegant body). Yes, it is true that men were known to faint when she walked into a room in a glamorous style generally reserved for storied Hollywood royalty. Don't be fooled, though, dear readers: She was no silly sexpot with a silly little head in the clouds. J was *hard* headed smart, well educated, and strong-willed to the max. On the soft side, she had an addiction to High Romance—a lust not just for men but for life. She lived it at full intensity—working exciting, high-level jobs in glam fields, sailing the Aegean. A great good sport, she was just as happy playing first mate or polishing brass as being pampered guest—and burning through the wicks on both ends of her candle.

After graduating from college, J applied to the Pinkerton National Detective Agency, the first step, as she saw it, to achieving her dream of becoming a spy. In those days, it was rare for a woman to apply for a "man's" job, but, as I said, J was rare. To her dismay, she discovered that Pinkerton was a rigidly "traditional" (code for sexist) organization and didn't allow even a well-trained female detective ("spy-in-training") to carry a gun. Guns were for members of the boys' club. The Pinkertons assigned J and the rest of the "girls" only low-risk, low-level surveillance assignments. Like a dime-store P.I., she'd sit in her car outside the office of a doctor suspected of cheating on his taxes, armed with a clicker-counter, not packing heat. Or she'd be asked to follow married men whose client wives suspected them of cheating. (One can only imagine the thrill she felt tailing these adulterous schlumps.) Meanwhile, the Pinkerton male rookies got to go on mob stakeouts and other dangerous jobs that would have fulfilled J's desperate craving for the dangers and thrills of a romantic, cinematic life in espionage.

Frustrated, furious, and disgusted by the rampant male chauvinism of the time, J turned high heel and left Pinkerton, never to look back. That's our backstory.

The scene of the crime in this story is J's glamorous penthouse in Midtown Manhattan—a single girl's dream pad, just steps from Bloomingdale's and her favorite swank bars. It was decorated like a richly decadent Moroccan paradise with a vast terrace for sunning and cocktail parties overlooking the bright lights of the big city. Then there was her bedroom. It was washed in all white tones with a king-size cloud bed, sumptuous ivory carpeting, and a bulb-lined, mirrored makeup table fit for Monroe's dressing room. It also had a grand closet with racks of couture clothing and flowing peignoirs. (J's good friend in the neighboring penthouse was national sales manager for Oscar, and he loved costuming our J, who dressed as she lived, ready always for high drama and romance.)

Now, sit back and imagine an old black-and-white Hollywood movie set. A glamorous bedroom designed for the studio's million-dollar star. There's a slow fade-out from the scene . . .

And then it happened. My mother, sitting at work, heard the phone ring and answered . . .

"K, I have something important to tell you. We must meet for lunch, *today!*"

"Must it be lunch, J? Just tell me now."

"I can't. Something has happened and I cannot discuss it over the phone."

The phone line crackled with tension from J's end.

They met at a ritzy hotel in Midtown, in a large lunchroom with widely spaced tables, so that J, safe from eavesdropping diners and bored, hovering waiters, could begin to tell her story.

The night before, J was asleep in her cloud bed in one of her summer-white nightgowns. Her straight, beautifully cut strawberry-blond hair was in perfect form, even in slumber: the picture of an angel at rest.

That is, until she stirred slightly, suddenly feeling, as she put it, "a presence in the dark."

She felt the presence of a man.

With the stunning apprehension of an intruder in her room, she opened her eyes and—instantly—a man's hand gently but firmly clamped over her mouth. Startled, she tried to jerk up but the man straddled her on the bed and carefully held her down with his superior male weight and strength. She said that in the dark she could make out only that he looked young—thirties maybe?—and had refined features, dark eyes, midlength hair, and a lean firm body: a handsome stranger holding her down in the dark.

He spoke in a slow, oddly reassuring, deep, manly voice: "Don't scream. I'm not going to hurt you. You just must be quiet. There's a reason I'm here and I have questions."

There was something about his calm demeanor and presence (as well as the confident tone of his voice) that was pleasant as well as disarming. Despite being initially alarmed, she did not feel endangered. He explained in a soothing yet stern manner that he worked for the CIA, in this mission, on behalf of the IRS, and that her father (who happened to be the head of the tax department for the western division of a major U.S. corporation) had discovered a blockbuster tax loophole with potentially disastrous repercussions to the country's vital revenue stream—costs to the government that could run into the billions. He was sleuthing for the CIA in their effort to determine if her father was working alone, and in the best interests of his company, or for a foreign state or entity.

In any case, the CIA and IRS had to put a stop to it!

Her head was spinning with the knowledge that the intruder knew her father's profession and position. But how? Was all this true? Was any of it true? It might be. She had to hear more.

Her thin frame relaxed a bit under the commanding pressure of his toned body and with the deliberate presentation of what to J appeared a seasoned operative. His hand remained in place over her mouth, and it was far more comfortable to listen than to struggle.

"I have gone through your filing cabinet and taken your business documents. We are expecting to find information that may help spell out your father's intentions. I have also found your rifle, chained and padlocked in your closet. I will leave it there. The pistol I found in your bathroom vanity I am taking so that you cannot shoot me."

J's father, an NRA member and the classic American stand-up guy, had trained J as a teenager to be a skilled markswoman and had given his only daughter a small, pearl-handled pistol for protection when she moved to New York.

The increasingly appealing intruder then slipped off of her and removed his hand, as gracefully as a panther, and asked her to open her safe. Inside were a gold Piaget watch and other fine jewelry and a few thousand dollars in cash—compliments of an older former lover, super-rich, insistently generous, estranged but not divorced from a wife who'd strayed—so his gifts to J were in the form of cash and jewelry—no checks, no paper trail. (An honorable man, when wifey had become seriously ill, he'd taken her back and, feeling remorse, left J the hefty nest egg that was now in her safe. Knowing that proudly independent J would refuse such a gift, he'd discreetly tucked it into an envelope marked "Mad Money" and hidden it in her travel bag of cosmetics.)

"Lie back down on the bed," the intruder demanded.

She did.

He tied her hands behind her head with rope from his pocket.

"I'm going to take items from your safe as assurance that you will not contact your father. If you do, the items will not be returned to you, and he may get hurt. This is a very serious matter for both agencies. The rope is loose enough that you can get out of it, but it will take you some time."

J nodded in compliance. As he was about to leave, he looked at her with lustful eyes, and she admitted to being scared but turned on as well.

"I want to make love to you," he said, fire in his eyes.

He set her pearl-handled pistol on the bedside table and took her without mercy, her delicate long limbs tied over her head. Bound and helpless, she was made love to passionately, for a long time (hours, J ardently reported).

Fade to black . . .

"So he raped you!" my mother flatly declared.

"Well, I guess you could say that. But he was so sexy and had such a firm body—he smelled so good!—that I didn't feel raped, K, I loved it," J admitted, more True Confessions than shamefaced confessional.

"I cannot believe that you fell for this guy's story, J! You must call your father *and* report this to the police," my mother insisted, rolling her eyes and resisting the urge to shout. (Could this have really happened?!)

"I can't! He knows so much, what if there's a possibility that it's real?" J continued, "I'm seeing him tomorrow. He said he's going to pick me up in a cab and make 'runs.' He is delivering payoff money to underground informants on the CIA payroll."

And so it continued.

J spent the next night willing the phone to ring, that ghastly familiar waiting game women play after a promising first date, the mind a crazy-making roller-coaster ride veering between high hopes and abject despondency.

Then. He called!

No private-sector traces in those pre–caller ID days.

J was swept off by her new, strange and stranger lover, watching enthralled from the taxi as he made his covert rounds, darting in and out of nondescript storefronts all around downtown and midtown Manhattan. She overheard his words of farewell, uttered in several different languages with the brio and casual assurance of—gasp! swoon!—an honest-to-goodness spy. At last J was living the exhilarating real-life adventure she was born to live, with an agent-operative on the upright-cowboy side of truth and justice. She anxiously awaited the resolution of the investigation into the business affairs of her Mr. Right Stuff daddy, his dossier being officially sealed and stamped CITIZEN ABOVE SUSPICION, as she knew him to be.

Thereafter, J's spy-lover would call her on random nights—always at night—and would also show up unannounced, at unexpected times. Their wild sexual affair became wilder and sexier during each clandestine rendezvous, as her romantic imagination continued to supersize the daring profile of her mystery man.

Then, the calls stopped.

Dead cold.

J began to get uneasy and angry, increasingly (if belatedly) suspicious of the whole story. He'd never sworn "Forever Darling," but he had sworn to return all the "borrowed" jewelry and cash.

No calls for weeks.

Raging silence.

My mother seized the moment to suggest—more like insist—that J contact a mutual old friend of theirs who just happened to be a tough, hardass NYPD detective we'll call A. In response to my mother's sensible idea, J relented, as she trusted that A would keep the matter private and not alert the NYPD without her consent. As they were to learn, A at the time was working undercover in Brighton Beach, a member of a team charged with infiltrating the Russian mob.

A arrived at J's apartment the next night. He was steely and solid, if restlessly on edge. His blue eyes fierce and foxlike, piercing right through cant and crookery, he was sharper than sharp. Here was her *real* James Bond, the recent former lover quickly becoming a Bond supervillain.

About one and a half minutes into J's story, A snarled his piece: "J, you're f'ing crazy. The guy's a scumbag." Shocked, and likely chagrined by his snap assessment, J agreed to A's plan to set up the scoundrel.

"Invite him over for a drink the next time he calls."

"What if he doesn't call . . . ?" J wondered aloud.

"He'll call. He'll come, and on his way out, carefully lift his glass with a cloth so we can dust for prints."

J agreed and found herself helplessly attracted to this latest caper, a new chapter with a new hero, a protective knight come to rescue the damsel.

One evening after work, J was unwinding and settling in for a rare evening at home when, as A had predicted, the phone rang, like a siren in the night.

It was him.

Finally, spy time! That bigger-than-Pinkerton spy moment J had been waiting for her entire life was about to unfold. Following A's instructions, J invited her target to come up for a drink. Then, taking a deep breath, she psyched herself for the performance of her life. She knew that her dark passenger/lover, like the detective, like an ace poker player, had a catlike sixth sense, and if there were any show of contrivance, he surely would detect that something was up. She must outfox him.

Would she? Could she?

Fearing harm if he caught on to the setup, J kept her cool.

Upon his arrival, J gave him a quick peck on the cheek and solicited his drink order, as she'd customarily done on previous visits. She purposefully showed a bit of peevish chill with her sarcastically dropped innuendoes about his abrupt "leave of absence." She intended to project hurt feelings, and his response told her it had been a smart ploy. As she handed him the Scotch glass (daintily held by the rim), he tugged it from her (attaboy! give me the whorls of all four fingertips, and the thumb—*yes!*), took a quick sip, set the glass down on the bar, and swept her back to the "scene of the crime" and a spirited reenactment of his amorous opening performance.

After lovemaking and pillow talk, she saw him to the elevator, watched him press the lobby button, and coyly blew him a kiss as the doors closed. She flew like hellfire back into her apartment, gently picked up the glass from the bar—using a cloth as A had instructed—and locked it away in the safe. The following day, the detective picked up the glass and put it into a plastic case. Two weeks later he called J to share his findings.

She was nervous, heart aflutter. Who was this secret lover?

"J, he's a grifter, a thief . . . the guy's got a long rap sheet, since he's nineteen, misdemeanors to low-grade felonies—up to this point—did some time as a juvie." A told her the man's real name and said that B, the name he'd given her, was one of many aliases.

He handed J a picture from the NYPD database of the attractive thief, on the street, wearing blackout sunglasses on his chiseled outlaw face, his thick black hair unruly. A surveillance shot from a few years back. The guy had been MIA ever since. A told her to try to set him up one more time so they could grab him.

He never called again.

J told the detective that she still couldn't figure out how he'd gotten into her apartment, as she had the best double-lock system, and there was no sign of damage to the hardware. On the night of the break-in, she'd asked the thief himself how he'd soundlessly gotten into her apartment, and he'd responded, "The Agency has tricks. I can get in anywhere."

New Years Eve 1979.

My parents were headed to a New Year's Eve bash at J's penthouse. They entered the elevator along with another couple, a dark-haired handsome man with a gorgeous blond girl in tight jeans and a faded leather jacket—not NYE party clothes. Curious, my mom stared at the man and then froze. She recognized him from the NYPD picture J had showed her. His eyes scanned and registered her reaction, and my mother could tell he knew that she knew. Coolly, he pressed the button for the very next floor, and the couple, without breaking a sweat, slipped off at the decoy floor, the girl following the man without any discernible reaction. A few floors later, the elevator stopped and the doors opened . . . to an empty hallway. The doors closed, and the elevator continued to the penthouse floor.

"J, you are *not* going to believe this!" K blurted out the instant J opened the door.

"What-what?" J stammered.

"I just saw your *man*, J."

"What-what-what . . . ?" J responded, suddenly grasping the message.

She raced to get the photo of him and ended up running down the stairwell, as the elevator was stalling with the entry of party-ready tenants on every other floor.

Entering the lobby, J shoved the picture in the doorman's face. "Have you seen this man?"

"You mean B?" the doorman calmly answered, calling the thief by what J knew was an assumed name. "Yes, he just walked out with his girlfriend."

"Do you *know* him?" J pressed on.

"Yeah, they lived in apartment ___. Their lease is up tomorrow. They turned in their keys as they left." (Note: The doorman tagged the apartment, but my mother can't recall the number.)

With the knowledge that the crime had been an "inside job," it was a snap for the detective to deduce that it hadn't taken a seasoned pro (though to J, her "spy" had seemed to be that) to gain access to her penthouse. Maybe he'd had the vixen accomplice distract the doorman while he pinched J's extra apartment key from the lobby mailroom, then managed to return it the same evening, as the doorman had never reported her key missing from the rack. A helped J file a police report and guided her in claiming tax deductions for all the stolen items. (Ha! The IRS took a small hit after all!)

Later in life, recounting events, J told my mother that the escapade with her criminal lover had been "the most thrilling and unforgettable experience of my life and the best sex I ever had" (and she had a lot of sex). "I don't regret it happening. He was a fantastic lover. So, okay, he's a thief. That's what he is. That's what he does."

J admitted that she'd also developed a serious crush on the guy wearing the White Hat, the detective A, and that he'd featured in a sexy Crime and Punishment scenario that played out in her fantasies for a long time.

End scene.

HOWEVER ONE MAY JUDGE J'S PRAGMATIC philosophizing, I, for one, give her the right to choose her own take on events. Certainly, no one can second-guess her verdict on the ecstasy of great sex—unexpected, racy, and electrified by an intoxicating whiff of the forbidden.

The story is offered merely to help stimulate your imagination in hatching potboiler plots for your own erotic story. I leave it to a Frenchman (in this case, Sartre) to best nail down the wisdom of our need for play: "We must act out passion before we can feel it."

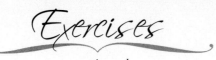

Exercises

continued

3. Pick a period of downtime during the day—perhaps the lull before lunch hour, or midafternoon, or right before bed—and for the next two weeks, at that exact same time, fixate on your erotic role-play scene. Even one-minute sessions will further charge your imagination and your appetite for indulgence.

4. Either masturbate to your own erotic story thoughts or imagine them as you're close to orgasming during sex. This will drive your passion for the real deal, whenever you choose to initiate play.

Okay, Posh Girls, let's get shady!

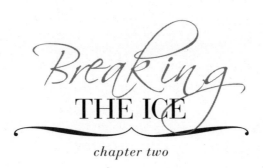

Breaking
THE ICE

chapter two

"**M**ost males are raised to think it's never okay to be rough with a woman," a male reader commented in a recent issue of *AskMen* magazine. By nature or nurture, the men we know are not Christian Greys, who, if you recall, had "issues" (damaging childhood = emotional wounds = intimacy issues). So, most of us have some work to do. A few key (if cliché) phrases that you should brand into your mind up front, as you prepare to approach your partner: "easy does it"; "one step at a time"; "haste makes waste"; and "be forthright but enchantingly so, with an overlay of mystery." Most importantly, own the thought that "all men are boys." It's our job to comfort and *keep 'em under control. *Wink.*

How to approach your partner and draw him into this new thrilling role play? By first developing and then communicating a solid understanding of what you want and don't want. It's time to engage your skills of persuasion and to act on your Wish List. Speaking of which, when's the last time you watched *Gone with the Wind*? For an awesome and stylish tutorial in the art of getting your way, it's hard to beat Miz Scarlett and her breathtaking arsenal of feminine wiles. Mr. H and I are both so crazy about that notion, in fact, that we recommend this: In any new or sticky situation, channel your Inner Belle and ask yourself, "What would Scarlett do?" (WWSD? for short—a running refrain scattered as a trigger jolt throughout this guide).

Ask Yourself Some Questions

What exactly does dominant/submissive role play entail, and which variations of play might a new initiate explore? Do you wade in with water wings and save the high-dive pyrotechnics for an older (maybe by a few days), wiser you? In this chapter, I'll be providing steps and hints to negotiating the terrain in this Edenic playland.

The very first step is to discover what type of caper you might like to try. How are you ever to know what you're looking for, what you're comfortable with, unless you give it a workout in your imagination? With that in mind, I offer you the First Commandment of DSRP: Let your id be your guide. Tamp down that bothersome superego and tap into your roiling, subconscious dream world to bring all those repressed feelings and desires out to play. Pick a favorite fantasy, romp around with it in your mind, study it, and make it your own. To begin, let's wheel in the Posh fantasy rack and let you pick through to select those you fancy. Being a naughty Posh girl, I want the whole rack, naturally. We'll start with the most popular, from the ready-to-wear rack, and progress to the haute couture fantasies.

Fancy the feel of the high-class call girl being ravaged and "taken" for his pleasure (channeling Julia Roberts and her powerful, dominant man in *Pretty Woman*)?

What about the damsel in distress, pleading for help from the big, strong, take-control guy who overpowers you sexually but also stands tall as your fierce protector (sounds like a job for the darkly mysterious masked swordsman Zorro)?

Perhaps the girl seized by the more physically aggressive soldier or the criminal rogue, recently freed from jail and ready to take you, after years of celibacy, like a beast crazed by hunger?

How about the posh, spoiled-brat starlet who needs training and punishment: being slapped, having her nipples pinched and her hair pulled to make her a good, submissive girl for her man?

Or maybe the haughty rich girl who is pleasantly horrified by the hot young stable-boy brute defiling her and "forcing" her to engage in unladylike sexual acts (my personal favorite)?

Wel-l-l-l, I like them all, I confess.

After you've thought through some possible scenarios, ask yourself what kind of actions might appeal to you. Having only your hands tied? Having your legs tied apart as well? Submitting to a full-body hogtie in which you are helpless and vulnerable to his every dirty sexual whim? Having a scarf tied about your mouth? Having your panties stuffed into your mouth? Would you like to be blindfolded or not? Choose from the manhandling menu of aggression levels: light, medium, or full-bodied? How about integrating some friendly sex toys? (Or does that ick you out?)

The first and most important step is to choose your ideal fantasy, starring your ideal dominant male character or behavior type—that, or build your fantasy around the guy who's already in your life and mold him to your specs. The nitty-gritty details are yours to discover, mull over, and opt for as you continue reading this guide.

SECOND STEP TO BREAKING THE ICE:
Figure Out What You *Don't* Want
Think deeply and creatively about all the things you might wish to enjoy, and then identify which types of role-play actions are *not* for you. Determine where your boundaries lie and set them in stone. Personal turn-offs, for example, might include aggressive, mean-spirited, merciless, or ruthless cruelty, or being hurt past your kink limits. Violence should *not* be part of the scene and, certainly, there should be

no infliction of serious injury. You may, however, reject the reverse: hesitancy, softness, a clear show of distaste.

As you make your decisions about behaviors that don't appeal to you, try to foresee the potential for triggering phobic reactions. You don't need to risk finding yourself unexpectedly uncomfortable with his strict commands and punishments. And you don't need to wait till he breaks out of the scene with everyone in gear, uneasy about what he perceives as nothing short of rape-commanding your love. Let me say this: These crises don't have to happen and can be headed off, or at least overcome, with a bit of preparation and basic training.

For example, maybe being constrained, fully tied up, handcuffed, or subjected to any sort of bondage isn't for you. How do you feel about being gagged? (I, for one cannot stand anything that inhibits, or threatens to inhibit, my breathing). Sexual toys like vibrators, cuffs, and paddles are also question marks—yea or nay? Do you want to be slapped? What I might say here, in reassurance and in encouragement of the spirit of adventure, is that there are many women who enjoy constriction and restraint, calling it "liberating" and saying it adds to their arousal and enhances the whole sexual experience. I must add, however, that comfortably submitting to such moves requires a strong degree of trust between parties; also, that bilateral trust strengthens relationships. Frequently, fears stem from overstepping preset limits of pain and humiliation, *and those fears are warranted.* In the world of DSRP, it is always best to trust your gut.

Once you've sorted all this out—remember, this is to be *your* movie, with you in the starring role!—you're *nearly* ready for the casting couch, that is, step three: recruiting your costar and selling him on the project. But right now—and this is important—let the word *limits* hover as loudly and clearly as a bothersome mosquito, right above all your thinking and planning. Keeping things "safe, sane, and consensual" is, for good reason, the mantra of BDSM and DSRP practitioners whose play does not constitute abuse. The actual setting of limits is the subject of the next chapter, and the only reason it doesn't lead off this guide (in flashing neon lights!) is because our initial focus is on the presentation of options central to the preplanning stages.

Communicate with Your Partner Using Basic Body Language and Demeanor

Back to *Gone with the Wind.* Is there a sexier, more romantic onscreen moment than when an enraged Rhett Butler sweeps Scarlett O'Hara off her feet and hauls her up the staircase to reclaim his rights to the marital bedchamber? Like a child throwing a show tantrum, Scarlett pounds her tiny fists feebly, halfheartedly on his manly chest. Did any of us believe for a second that Scarlett really, *really* meant to rebuff her long-spurned, reinvigorated husband, emboldened by alcohol to stop with all the Southern chivalry and challenge his willfully misguided wife? Not even for a split second. And whom did we cheer for? Not for the husband, not for the wife, but for the two of them—the star-crossed couple.

Women knew, they just knew, that Rhett's fed-up, lust-filled rage had to be a turn-on to his headstrong wife, determinedly celibate since giving birth and losing her eighteen-inch waistline. We knew, didn't we, that what Scarlett was really saying was "Let's play," and "Take me, take me, Rhett. I will act horrified as you rip off my petticoat. I will feign outrage as you ravage me like the hungry, bloodthirsty beast that you are." But Mr. Clark Gable, er, Rhett, sees right through her girly "don't take me/take me" sexually frustrated body language and does . . . what comes naturally.

So who had his/her way with whom? The answer is clear, I believe, to any red-blooded woman, and if you need a reminder, revisit the scene on YouTube (search "Scarlett O'Hara Rhett staircase"). If you can say that's not an Oscar-winning self-satisfied look of guilty pleasure on Scarlett's face as she luxuriates on the morning after in her Southern belle featherbed, then Miss Vivien Leigh won her Academy Award without your vote.

I give the pride of early placement to this iconic scene from *Gone with the Wind* because, to me, it's the essence of what DSRP should be: fun, romantic, passionate, intense, and liberating. We have much to learn from it . . .

How do we use body language hints in bed to get him to play the dominant? Simple gestures at first: try crossing your arms over your head as if they were tied. Speak the words "hold me down." This can progress to your saying, "Why don't you get your tie or my stockings and tie my hands? I want to feel like I can't escape from you." As he's taking off your panties, kick and fight like someone new to sex. Now that the games have begun, he'll read that not as defensive but as a playful act of defense or aggression, which will embolden him to get tougher with you. Score! Scratch, nip, bite, tug at his hair in a childlike way, summoning just a bit of the rage of Scarlett's girly temper tantrum, so he gets the unmistakable message that this is an invitation for him to "discipline you" and to take charge. We've all heard the cliché "men need to be trained"—so train his arse!

Body language is a powerful tool for breaking the ice: a nonthreatening way to communicate and manipulate your partner into giving you what you want in order to indulge your fantasies. Yet unlike our spontaneous younger selves, as adults we have accepted the social conditioning that trains us to carry ourselves in a stiff manner, to be always in control. As youngsters, we let our emotions dictate our body language. We kicked, bit, thumped our fists, went into the fetal position, stuck out our tongues—we *let go*, let it all out. It was innate behavior, simple, straightforward, and, surely you recall, most effective. Youngsters are extremely fluent when it comes to body language, and while adults see this as evidence of "immaturity," it's actually the purest form of human expression, untainted by social norms and by what we feel to be "correct."

Consider this: In bed, conduct is private. So get rid of that stiff stuff, let your guard down, and lose that restrictive social conditioning! Tap into your pure youthful behavior and show your partner what you want by relearning to express that early body language. Expressing your desires nonverbally, giving hints about what you want and don't want through relaxed, freed-body behavior in bed is such an easy and natural way to communicate with your partner. It lets you get what you want (*your* way) by giving him what he wants (his way). Go for it!

By way of example of how body language can ease him into play, let me share with you a kinky tale.

I was having dinner at Elaine's (a virtual institution on Manhattan's Upper East Side, popular with writers, publishing world execs, and Woody Allen, sadly now shuttered with the recent death of its irreplaceable namesake proprietor) with a flame, then one of the senior executive editors at the *New York Times*. He was older, and while down-to-earth and an easy conversationalist, he broadcast a powerful "I'm the boss" demeanor. Dressed in pinstripes, he was an old-school Brooks Brothers study in intellectual elitism. He wasn't stuffy, however, no blowhard social conservative, and our personas overlapped on the outré edges, drawing us together as lovers. That night, after sharing small talk with a slew of tony reporters, writers, and some celebs who'd swung by our table to say hi (to him, that is), we breezed off in the rain. I remember that I had an umbrella with a broken spoke and that it didn't cover both of us. He characterized the busted umbrella as having a "poetic flaw." Almost a metaphor for what was to come, as I waaaay surprised him with some wild and kinky action, which luckily he saw as poetic and not flawed.

We spoke as equals (I'm pretty good with the spoken word, even when I'm outclassed), and, in fact, I was turned on by his power, stature, solid presence, and mature, brilliant mind. I had an urge for him to ravage me, but I could sense that he wore his pinstripes to bed. Maybe it was the tempest outside the window, the primal resonance of rain nailing the earth, that got me into a wild state when we arrived. Whatever it was, I started to roughhouse with him, pushing a bit, play wrestling, and he responded playfully. Our roughhousing escalated and I—oooops!—gave him a girly sock to the face. He pinned me up against the wall and well,

Paid. Me. Back. But good! In a very controlled, almost Germanic way—not as a wild and hungry beast but certainly dominating me—he let me know who now was in charge, that I had no say. Through calculated body language, I'd projected that provocation, and subjugation was the state I wanted to inhabit, and he caught on, performing masterfully.

The next day, I met him at the *New York Times* offices, as we had a preplanned date for him to show me around the building. I exited the elevator and saw a glaring shiner on his right eye. OMG. But he kept cool and walked me through the rows of writers typing away, proudly showing off a recently hung artist's collage of actual *New York Times* front pages. We slipped into his big impressive office, floating way above the rows of worker bee desks. Now alone, we kissed and he said, his eyes all lit up and dancing, "I have never had an experience like that before. I have never *done* anything like that before!" He said he'd been making up excuses for the black eye all day long. Ha! I'll confess it was more than a little amusing to see all the writers, reporters, and junior editors running around below, never imagining that the petite blond in the black sundress had been the one to give the mighty boss a black eye. We laughed about it, and I certainly wasn't made to feel there was any cause for apology. On the contrary, he exuded pride and residual pleasure over our kinky-rough dominant/submissive tango.

You see, through his show of overpowering male sexual dominance, he had ended up having his way with me, so I choose to see things as an eye for an eye. *Wink.

Tra la laaaa . . . moving on.

FOURTH STEP TO BREAKING THE ICE:
Use Language to Approach the Subject of Indulging Your Fantasies
You might start by telling him (lures best dangled at bedtime), "I'm going to share a fantasy: I'm a [fill in your chosen role-play identity] and you are a [fill in your fantasy male character]."

Or, "I have my hands tied, and I want to hear you say: 'This can hurt, or, if you're good, I won't hurt you.'"

Or, "Pretend I'm your prisoner."

(WWSD?)

If it becomes clear that he's uneasy or flat-out turned off by your being so forward, or, in other words, if you sense that he just feels it isn't "right" to be physically aggressive or dominating to a woman, then . . .

Cut to the fallback part of your plan, telling him that this is your erotic fantasy, that although he may see it as "dirty play," it is not abuse in tonight's playbook because you are inviting it, *willing* it. He's a good guy, he respects and shows respect for women—that's why you love him! But . . . not tonight, dear. Show me some spunk!

You're verbally drawing him into irresistibly titillating territory here, and once you've lured him in, you can start things off by getting physical with playful slaps, pinches, hair-tugging, lightly aggressive actions delivered as if in jest while giggling or otherwise showing that this is all in the spirit of a rousing good romp. This will let him know it's okay to slap, pinch, and return your sexy provocations, responding with the same strength levels you exhibited with him. At that point, you can allow things to escalate to your comfort levels of intensity and scope, taking both of you to the next level of play (described in subsequent chapters).

Overcoming a Roadblock

If your man is just not having it, no matter what you say or do, there is a problem. It's not you, and it shouldn't be too hard for you to solve. The fear is inside him, as the majority of men (even the most controlling rough cowboy or SOB business tycoon) ice up when first invited to dominate a bit in bed, i.e., outside their professional arena. Might you have a secret submissive male? Statistically, it's not likely. In my interlude as a pro dominatrix, I saw very few men turn out to be secret submissives.

And of those, I'd say that 75 percent—even the wimps—were, instead, "switch" players, the S&M world's term for those who like to play it both ways. Very few men wish to be exclusively submissive.

So, assuming your man is not a secret submissive, what's his problem?

There are countless possible psychological reasons for his hesitation. Did he suffer an abusive childhood? Was he reared in a very religious household with clear-cut sexual taboos? Has he elevated you to an impossibly high pedestal? For the purposes of this guide, let's bypass all that, because troubleshooting the root of such misgivings (not to mention the cure) may take a lifetime. There are easier routes.

Most men are into one sport or another, so, to advance one approach to overcoming your man's reluctance, polish up your gamesmanship. By giving your S&M fantasies a sporty theme, you shift emphasis from shady shenanigans to familiar games, moves, and fields. You can start with a friendly arm wrestling match—a physical fighting competition that he knows to be cute and harmless, which will lead to fun and laughter. Then take things further. Try wrestling with him, an activity weighted in his favor and sure to end with his muscling you into a position of submission. Sports-themed rituals also stir up his competitive instinct to "play to win."

Another friendly game: Taunt and playfully make fun of him. Pick a fight. Make him jealous by talking favorably about another man (now there's a ploy straight out of Scarlett's playbook!). Laugh and gently ridicule him if he gets something wrong and say, "It's so annoying when you do [whatever]." But keep it light; don't go for the jugular. In an agitated state, he'll take out his frustration on you with aggressive hot sex—no wonder they say that make-up sex is the best! Once this dynamic is initiated, he'll take to the act more willingly the next time you have sex, and that's when you can "fight back" a bit, letting him slip naturally into retaliatory mode himself. Remember, men don't forgive physical provocation as easily as women do, and they have more trouble articulating their frustrations. In other words, you can count on him to reciprocate, once the game gets going.

Talk About It

Have a couple of dainty drinks, and then read him a few of the tastiest paragraphs of *Fifty Shades*. Download a film: *Secretary, Blue Velvet, In the Realm of the Senses* (beautiful, erotic, mesmerizing cinema from Japan, though you may want to hit the off button before sexual obsession leads to, ummm, the mistress's snuffing of her lover's , uhhh, manhood). While watching the movie, react emotionally to the tough love, and afterward, try telling him that you felt ambivalence about the freaky stuff. That, yes, you found it freaky but that, surprisingly (getting your fox on), you also found it kind of . . . hot.

You might also mention that many of your girlfriends are trying this "role-play stuff" and that it's made you curious to know what all the fuss is about. Improvise, be engaging, use whichever words you feel will best ease him into it. The next day, try texting him a bondage photo from the web, commenting, "Ha!" (Google image-search "bondage photos" for choices ranging from the high-fashion art of Helmut Newton to the decidedly less tasteful). Email him an article on S&M, how "everybody's trying it" since the release of *that book* . . . can you believe it?!¹ And so on. Discuss these teasing gestures later, registering suitable shock but adding, "Well, it might be fun . . . I don't know. I think I might like to try it?" (Time for a sheepish grin.) Cultivate coyness, or whichever approach is your usual standby for expressing something hard to say. (WWSD?) For many men, a woman acting girly, coquettish, or even bashful can be a turn-on. It makes them feel in control, and here your guy may take the ball and run, co-opting your new idea and calling it his own. And remember, you don't have to be a spring chicken to act *chicky*. Look at the French chicks!

If you're lucky enough to have a man who likes a forward woman, you can skip the preliminaries. Lay on your fantasies, and start with the racy suggestions. Boom. Done. Ice broken . . . and into the fire. But first, you must map your road to desire.

A POTENTIAL SNAG, REPORTED BY "MY man on the street."

During the writing of this guide, a union chief in New York City—a friend of my Posh Guide male contributor, Mr. H—called me, rather astonished, to relate a conversation he'd overheard among a group of construction workers on a building site he was managing. Here was a pack of hardboiled hardhats, *talking about DSRP!* Wow. My eavesdropping reporter was particularly amused by one worker's characterization of his wife's demands: "She wants me to get all *romantic* and sh*t, put on a tie and pull her hair—that's scary . . . and what? I'm not good enough?" he added with a comedic, self-conscious guffaw. His coworker pals chimed in with their own "I hear yas," relating how their wives, too, were suddenly wanting to try role play. And yes, they fingered *that book* as the agitator.

Interesting development, I'd call it. With reverberations *everywhere*—in media reports, in advertising, and even in college curricula—in a culture jolted by a blockbuster bondage novel, here is street-level evidence that you and I and Cyndi Lauper aren't the only girls who want to have fun. From Europe to the United States, from urban professionals to suburban moms, Ivy League co-eds, and the wives of hardhats, women have spoken: We want to *P-L-A-Y!*

Okay, this is an encouraging state of affairs: a tsk-tsking society shedding its puritanical notions. But there may be a problem here. As the construction worker put it, "What? I'm not good enough [and here I finish the sentence with his unspoken words] for her?" Let's go there.

First: Anticipating such insecurities on the part of men made uneasy by the springing of "exotic," unconventional ideas, Mr. H and I set about updating his website, www.HIsfortheHunter.blogspot.com. It's an excellent forum of tutelage and coaching from him, comments and Q&A from his targeted male readers. The reader feedback makes it a rich source of information and feedback for you and me, which is the reason I sought his valuable guy-side insights for the *Posh Girl's Guide to Play*. In later chapters of this guide, as online, you'll see that, in advising men on both the basics and the fine points of DSRP, Mr. H coaches with the skill and finesse of a locker room pro. You may wish to use him as a resource, even, perhaps, as a stand-in for direct contact, if you're feeling uncomfortable in the proposing and teaching roles. Use him and this guide, in other words, to pick up where *that book* left you off: hungry to experience role play yourself but clueless about the pursuit. Judging from all the frustrated yearning I've been blog-reading, I'd say you're not alone.

So, then, how do we address the reactions of a man who is hurt or confused as to why you want to explore DSRP? A couple of hints: Don't get angry, but at the same time, don't let your empathy cause you to put a halt to your pursuit of a sideline sexual activity that may just sweeten your life as a couple.

Let's break it down: Admitting your wish to try DSRP may change your identity in his eyes. Because it's all you've communicated to him thus far, he understandably assumes that you are strictly vanilla-world straight in your sexual preferences—a missionary-position female uninterested in a new kind of erotic or playful sex. There is a psychological comfort for him in hanging on to this prevailing perception.

So why change it? Well, I think the brave decision to reveal your sexual fantasies (previously repressed or brand new) speaks to the primary aim of this book, which I see as nothing short of expanding women's freedom of choice: *granting ourselves permission* to experience liberation from every social convention that tells us how to be a good girl, wife, or lover. Allowing ourselves the freedom of sexual exploration may be the final frontier.

This brings to mind a big and relevant ponderable thought, attributed to Jean-Paul Sartre: "Freedom is what you do with what's been done to you." Which, in context, I tie to the expectation that we know ourselves and that our self-interest derives from self-esteem and self-respect, i.e., is not narrow, is not *purely* id-driven.

An important point is that if your partner can come to see your sharing of erotic fantasies with him as a new and exciting liberation for you, he is likely to be turned on by your passion and appreciate that it is a journey you are undertaking together. It's when a woman is sheepish or reserved about sharing her sexual fantasies, when she can bring herself to do nothing more than drop "hints," that her partner is likely to be confused and think there's something "wrong with him" as a sexual partner. Hints are okay as early-stage icebreakers, but confining communication to hints or half-assed suggestions usually signals bad news. It's important to be fully open and brave with your man, to entertainingly divulge (progressively, if that suits) the various sexual fantasies that excite you. He then can read your proposition for play as a fun challenge, an experiment, rather than as an insult to his manhood or sexual performance.

Perhaps you might read or relate to him the personal erotic tale I offered earlier in this chapter—the one featuring the *New York Times* editor. See what he makes of it. Ask if he can relate to the seductive (and successful!) initiation of a "good guy" into the macho world of DSRP. Does he relate positively? Then you're home free! Just as it happened in the tale, telling the story will build heat too—Posh Girl's promise!

Now, to round out the picture, let's get the guy's perspective on the subject of breaking the ice, starting with a lead-in maxim from Mr. H: "There is nothing sexier to a man than a sensually exciting woman who knows what she wants in the bedroom."

INTERVIEW WITH MR. H

Alexis: Can you expand on the wise ways a girl can reveal, approach, and execute her role-play appetites, after she's hinted at her interest in DSRP? Which approaches are likely to capture his attention and interest while ensuring her safety?

Mr. H: Well, that first step, telling your man about your interest in bondage and role play, is going to be a little nerve-wracking, but if you go in prepared, it should be a relatively painless process. We men are eager but socially programmed toward chivalry, you know, doing the honorable thing in our romantic interactions with women.

Most men have their own bondage/role play–related fantasies, but many struggle with the element of aggression. We've been reared to stay away from what might be perceived as *actual* aggression toward women. [Author's note: In performance, permissible fantasies rely not on *real* aggression but instead on the illusion of aggression, but that's a detail we'll play around with later in this guide.] For many men, shifting from the secret fantasies of bondage and role play to the reality—without *your* help in getting them there—is a transition they secretly wish to make but they do so with difficulty, having to reorder their programmed qualms in order to take a strong, "aggressive" tack on sexuality and fantasy.

Alexis: For many of us, of both sexes, DSRP is a new frontier, but I should think that once we women steel ourselves to "pop the question," our men's eyes would light up, like kids at the candy counter. Please let us in on some thoughts likely to pass through a guy's mind as he works through his partner's proposal and realizes, "Hey, she's talking her and me!"

Mr. H: In my travels—real-world and online—through this wild world of fantasy, and in conversation with many women involved in DSRP (I did run a Q&A advice column back in the day), it sounds like a solid third of men approached will struggle greatly with this kind of role play *in the beginning*. On top of this, I would guess that there is a quarter who will never agree to engage in this kind of play (just as 25 percent of men say they wouldn't take a yoga class), for whatever personal or philosophical reasons. That leaves a "game" 40-plus percent primed to become *enthusiastically* game if their partner takes the reins and works with them to open their minds to notions they're already toying around with in the deep closets of their minds, when nobody is looking.

While your guy might have explored these fantasies in private, it's up to you, after expressing your interest, to make him feel safe about what you as a couple are about to explore. Many men may be warily suspicious that you are "testing" them or trying to see what kind of people they secretly are, so it's important to assure them that this isn't some new development reflecting your dissatisfaction with their performance in the bedroom. Your ability to clearly explain the what, when, and why will have a huge beneficial effect on how they progress in their earnest attempts to help you fulfill your needs.

Here are five key points to cover in your conversation with your man about your interest in exploring DSRP:

1. How long have you wanted to try this and why? For many men, an out-of-the-blue overture will register as cause for alarm. Your man may read it as the expression of a sudden need to spice up what he suspects must be a lackluster love life. It's up to you to tame these thoughts and let him know that this is "supplementary," that it will bare an aspect of your sexuality that he will get to explore with you, and that it will be a journey different and apart from your "regular" love life.

2. Do point out the current, growing popularity of this type of play scene. If a man suspects that your proposal is something way out of the ordinary, he may fear that he's being asked to entertain bizarre, out-of-bounds notions, and this may make him reluctant to consent.

3. Focus on the word *fantasy*. Many men haven't engaged their creative imaginations since childhood, and it's not always easy for them to flip the switch back on while struggling with the "reality" aspect. You can make them feel safe (and sound) in their "pretending" by encouraging it as a perfectly natural and promisingly enjoyable element of adult DSRP. I've received many emails from women struggling with comments like "I'll never hit a girl!" and "That just sounds too rough and mean, and I'm not mean to women!" which shows a fundamental misunderstanding of what's being asked of them. Make an effort to relay the amount of control that is involved and slowly teach them that, in truth, this is anything but a mad, chaotic pursuit. Rather, it will be staged as a carefully planned interlude in which each of you adopts a new role, indulging a shared fantasy (and exercising your unalienable right to the pursuit of happiness). If

they need time to adjust, give them time. Nothing is worse than pushing a new idea too quickly and coming on too strong.

4. Home in on your partner's specific fantasies and encourage his contributions in this direction from the get-go. The sooner he gets turned on by the conversation, the sooner he'll put his insecurities aside. I remember that when I first started to explore these kinds of scenes, the more I discussed my own ideas, the easier it became and the more confident I grew in trying them out. Coax your man into discussing his thoughts, interests, and feelings. You can take the driver's seat, while foxily allowing him to feel like the seat is his, by taking that little trickle of thought and turning it into a flood of fantasy.

5. Remind your man of the benefits. Make the conversation sexy. You don't want to be too clinical and detached, as it may go right over the head of a resistant partner. If you know how to seduce a man into the bedroom on a "normal" basis, the same tricks will work here, at least until you've tossed him the reins, at which point he'll be 100 percent in command of what happens. Put yourself in his shoes—new game, new rules, unfamiliar neighborhood, risky part of town—and you'll see that some reassurance is in order. Encouraging words alone can bust a lot of barriers and show him that you have confidence in his ability to "give it" and in your strength and commitment to "take it"—all for a good cause, of course.

   Getting your man to "play along" won't be an easy task in all cases, but why treat it any differently from any other difficult thing you've convinced your partner to do? As with anything he was reluctant to explore (vacationing in an exotic land, dining at a restaurant with no steak or pasta on the menu, meeting your straightlaced *father*), you need to focus on the rewards and let him know that he can play things his way. In present context, the typical "macho-defensive" statements of protest (e.g., "I'm not rough with girls") are made more out of insecurity, fear of failure, and a lack of knowledge than from actual dislike of the fantasy, so you'd be wise to work on taming those fears, while letting him know that you see this adventure as mutually gratifying and rewarding.

While some men are "born" to do this, if you feel that your man needs a helping hand to maneuver him into your fantasy of a dominant partner, venture the thought that DSRP will allow him to indulge all those superheroic youthful fantasies that are repressed by red-blooded adult men in our civilized modern world.

The more confident you are, and the more confident you make him feel, the more likely you are to take a hard-to-convince partner and have him convinced that he thought of it first. I'd know, because this is exactly how it went with me many years ago when I was wooed into my first role-play venture.

Alexis: And with that, I say take charge of your fantasy life and then let him take charge as your dominant play partner. It works! Do it! Spill it! Part of being a responsible adult male or female is putting on your big-boy pants or big-girl panties and dealing with those touchy, uncomfortable conversations that are sometimes necessary. In this case, the little trick to getting what you want is called "asking for it." Once you relay your wishes and fantasies to your lover, massive rewards are right around the corner.

Exercises

1. Imagine the various outcomes possible in sharing your fantasies and your interest in trying DSRP:

> *a. Indifference*
> *b. Ridicule*
> *c. Rejection*
> *d. Acceptance*

Prepare a calm, controlled, and positive response to the first three. Decide to be courteous, even if your talk turns into a disagreement. Concentrate more on the possibility of acceptance. It builds confidence.

Note: His first reaction may be negative, owing to a fear of something new. Do not get angry and do not take it personally. It simply means you have work to do, on him and maybe on your approach. Allow the idea to settle in, and give him time to accommodate the new within his set view of sex. A good bet is that he will be accepting but will want answers and direction. Tell him or simply send him the link to www.HIsfortheHunter .blogspot.com, our "for the boys" DSRP guide.

2. Recall a time when, even though it was difficult, you were compelled to confess something embarrassing—to a friend, foe, family member, coworker, lover, whomever. Ask yourself:

> *a. What did you think and feel before making your confession?*
> *b. What did you think and feel afterward? Were you relieved? Did you feel stronger?*

3. Place an empty chair in front of you and imagine your lover sitting in it. Envision his face, hair, eyes, the way he smells, the details of his clothing. This might take ten minutes. Then begin to read "him" your erotic DSRP story, or simply tell him about your interest in DSRP and touch on some of your fantasies. (You may recognize this technique—talking to an imagined partner—as one successfully employed by both therapists in session and method acting teachers in class.)

If you find yourself getting into it, you could do it a second time but with one difference. Put the different possible reactions listed above, in Exercise 1, in separate envelopes. Select one of the envelopes at random and put it on the chair. As you start talking about your interest in DRSP, or reading your story and touching on some of your DSRP fantasy actions, stop midway, then open the envelope and continue talking to "him" based on that reaction. Continue the exercise until you have responded to each reaction.

This might sound like a long-haul process, but it will not only build your confidence but also help you sort out how you will express your feelings without *hmmms*, *wel-l-l-ls*, and other awkwardness. Further, it will help tone down any possible angry, aggressive, combative, or hurt feelings that may surface if, initially, he's not fully accepting. You'll want to avoid a fight or, worse, a fear-based conviction that you must never share your sexual fantasies or interests again.

Besides, once the proverbial cat is out of the bag, you're not going to get her back in. If that's a scary thought, consider the scarier prospect of living the rest of your life "in the closet." Repressing your sexual feelings begins as annoyance and grows to a soul-crushing piece of degrading psychological baggage. Not a backpack you're going to enjoy hauling around, when you could unzip, open it up, toss out the dirty little secrets like so much confetti, and live! All you have to gain is a healthy, sexy, satisfying relationship.

And now to the *très très importante* chapter 3: Limits.

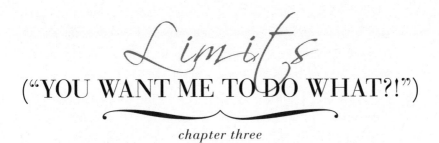

Limits
("YOU WANT ME TO DO WHAT?!")

chapter three

This just in! Harvard University (Harvard!) has officially recognized the Munch Club, which serves the school's S&M community (Harvard! BDSM!). Only thirty members so far, but that's up from seven in 2012, a 450 percent spike in a year. (Harvard! Bottoms up! Spank and be spanked!). And get this: They're ten years behind Iowa State University, where there's been a bondage club since 2003. Yes, dear readers, BDSM has come to the ivy-covered precincts of Cambridge and to the heart of the heart of the country, as the *New York Observer* reported in a front-page article titled "The Story of 'No': S&M Sex Clubs Sprout Up on Ivy Campuses, and Coercion Becomes an Issue."[1] "I've been hit with a riding crop, a belt, a paddle, canes, a flogger," a co-ed coos (anonymously). "Floggers are my favorite." The focus of the piece expands to include other Ivy League schools, where the reporter exposes big trouble in paradise, as "some young members . . . are finding the subculture is offering them more of an education than they expected, confronting them with serious issues involving consent, disclosure, anonymity, sexual violence, guilt and innocence, crime and punishment."

It happens. Shit happens. Even at Harvard. Let's not let it happen to you.

Introducing Limits

In this "me-first" chapter, I am going to present some concepts, define some important terms, and draw some useful distinctions. First off, DRSP is not a New Year's Eve party, where everyone dresses up, gets smashed, and goes wild. DSRP must not be a free-for-all bacchanal mess. Why? Because that's how submissives get hurt and the fun stops. As in every wildly exciting engagement between players, there are rules to the game. It's not just toss-your-dominant-a-crop-and-let-'em-ride. No. We will discuss the importance of communicating to your dominant both your physical and verbal limitations, your "hard" and "soft" limits, and your safe words and gestures prior to the kinky fun that is role play.

When preparing to explore the world of DSRP, it is up to you to determine your limits—to identify actions, words, and absolutely anything else related to sex play that makes you uncomfortable. In this chapter, I will categorically define limits and discuss the importance of deciding and declaring what's acceptable and what's to remain off-limits in your DSRP practices. In short, a "hard limit" refers to a no-no that is not up for debate or compromise—now or ever—with your play partner. A "soft limit" is a no-no *for now*—one that, at this pre-tryout stage, makes you mildly uneasy but could be subject to second thoughts and possible adoption into future play routines (*conditionally*, subject to *your* conditions).

Note: for a True Confessions account of unscripted, "anything goes" scene play gone disastrously awry (I was there), see the addendum at chapter's end.

Soft Limits

The gray area. You see room for "maybes" if your lover desperately wants to explore a soft territory action or path that you are not quite digging. Perhaps he'd like to see you in a saucy costume, to deliver some mildly punishing verbal taunts, or stage your play in the noirish shadows of a motel on the wrong side of the tracks (his hard-boiled private eye to your defenseless maiden). The point is that none of these propositions represent an egregious violation to your physical or mental well-being, nothing that sets off the flashing red X of a fight-or-flight response. Rather, while they aren't exactly to your taste, you reserve the right to mellow on that if they turn out to be hot-ticket important to your partner.

I, for example, am seriously claustrophobic and reject any mouth gags. If I feel I can't breathe, I start to panic. Mr. H, however, loves the visual image of a mouth gag. What to do? Well, we came up with a compromise solution. Through a tryout session, I discovered that I could accept a very loose-fitting scarf gag, providing enough wiggle-room that I didn't freak out, though tight enough to stay in place and give Mr. H his turn-on. Why did I compromise? I saw it as my gain if my partner was aroused, as he would be more into me and the play. Cue fireworks.

Let's say that your soft limit is hand-spanking, bondage, or a costume. Then, perhaps, he could spank lightly or only once during play. Or perhaps the bondage gear could be so loose that you can easily disengage. Still, the visual would be there for him. So you don't want to wear a fully themed costume? Consider instead accessorizing with just one or two pieces of the outfit—enough to trigger his fantasy visual, but not so costumey as to make you feel ridiculous.

First-time players, however, should think twice about compromising their soft limits. Things can escalate quickly and lead to sticky situations that could turn both of you off to further exploration into play. (Note: A little fender-bender needn't end the excursion; disaster recovery tips are coming up later in this chapter.)

Hard Limits

As a general rule, it's important that a hard limit remain an emphatic "No. Not going to happen, pal." You slap those hard limits down *hard*. They are not up for debate or compromise. And be sure to lay out your hard limits in detail. Clarity here is more important than a richly detailed spilling of fantasies. Trust me on this.

There may be room for take-it-backs, however, where you may consider allowing hard limits to tip into soft-limit territory. That said, your dominant *must* respect the fact that only you—*not* he—can make such a decision.

Sometimes, hard limits stem from social conditioning or irrational fears that hold a woman back, dictating thoughts and behavior on a subconscious level. Therapists liken them to the repressed and repressive boogeymen of an "unexamined life." That kind of life "isn't worth living," as everyone's favorite Greek uncle, Socrates, famously said at his trial for heresy. His crime: encouraging his students to challenge the accepted beliefs of the time and to think for themselves. For that, he got the death penalty, but, luckily for us, we're rocking to the tunes of the twenty-first century and aren't forced to choose between an unexamined life and death by hemlock. Refusing to take stock of our past and present has been likened to stumbling through life without a road map—and without a map, it's hard to determine our path and reach our destination, no? The remarkably awesome upside is that when you begin to know yourself, to take control of your life, it gives you the freedom to become the person *you* want to be.

Okaaaay, then, jumping off my Greek soapbox (couldn't resist—those wise old Athenian ancients had things all figured out, and they said it *so well!*), and back to kicking limits . . .

By way of strategic example, I throw out my own seemingly *organic* repulsion to BJs. So extreme that during an early, blink-of-an-eye marriage, I would refuse my husband's requests with the fuck-off line "go get a hooker." Years later, through my play experience with Mr. H, I started to analyze why I felt so repelled by this common sexual practice. It came to me that I saw it as degrading to women, namely me.

Gradually, gingerly taking baby steps into the, for me, new and wondrous world of DRSP, I found that (1) dishing it out as a pro domme hadn't prepared me for this role reversal, and (2) I was reacting to what felt like internal orders, being issued not in my voice but by unwelcome tyrants, voices superimposed on my own. They were the voices of taskmasters I'd heeded in childhood and internalized: my socially conservative parents, my girls' school teachers, and my classmates. In other words, the world I knew. Add that to my (congenital, I think) unhealthy extreme anger toward authority, and you get the picture: a carefully reared girl-child living pissed off by convention and yet unable, or unwilling, to pull away. My aversion to giving a BJ was coming from a place of social conditioning that whispered to me, "Ladies don't give BJs." (See what I mean? Silly, but that's what comes of being cruelly sheltered among one's own reticent caste.) As for my hostility to power sharing, both in and out of bed, I saw that it was just that: innate hostility, stubbornly played out in a self-sabotaging battle of the sexes. Further, I grew to recognize pride-based fears, products of my own insecurity and overblown feelings of vulnerability.

Once I confronted my qualms, my hard limit of no BJs shifted to the soft column: I would do it if and when I felt like it. I'll never be overly fond of giving my lover a BJ during play, but it excites me that I am able to do it and that, clearly, for him, it is a heaven-sent "gift." Personally, I've found BJs to be an unexpected turn-on, in that they may be the ultimate submissive act for me, letting me relax into sub-space.

Sometimes I like to pretend I hate a kinky action and say, "No, no, stop, no," but my partner Mr. H has known me for six years, and I can trust him to know when my actions and words *really* mean *no*. Obviously, such transgression demands serious-ass trust that your partner is alert and able to read your signals correctly. Ideally, the two of you have established a close relationship over a long period of time. Still, playing with hard limits is risky business, tipping toward edge play, which I hereby define.

Edge Play

This concept should be self-explanatory. It's risky, *not* for beginners, perhaps not for you, ever. In edge play, you and your partner, at some point beyond the initial foray into DSRP, mutually agree to cross your hard limit list. Suddenly there are no *no*s. Agreeing to let your dominant have full control over you, whether you like the commands and actions or not, can rouse excitement, as what formerly was illusion is now the real deal: Your wish no longer is his command, so it's all, "What's up next?" Edge play will be addressed in more depth in chapter 12, targeted *only* to advanced players. Even for that group, there are experienced DSRP players who discourage edge play. Please mull that thought if you're of a mind to skip ahead to chapter 12, and be warned: You'll be on your own, dancing on the razor's edge. I should point out that the discussion of edge play in chapter 12 stays in the guide because we will not discourage an adventurous pro if your gut tells you that (1) you can handle it and (2) you're partnered with a man who's earned your perfect (*unqualified*) trust. Still, we suggest guidelines and offer warning stories of ways edge play can go terribly wrong. In other words, we try to give it to you straight, yet leave the ultimate decision making to you.

If you do find yourself attracted to a hard-limit practice you've seen in an erotic movie or novel or perhaps heard about from friends, it's a sound idea to try it out through private fantasizing before proceeding to the real-world audition. Then, you may more reliably trust your gut as to whether or not you greenlight the project.

So, regarding hard limits, here's the message, in a nutshell: "Know thyself." (Just can't shake those Greeks!) That aphorism is engraved for posterity on the Temple of Apollo at Delphi, and it *deserves* to be engraved on a twenty-four-karat gold heart, with the flip side reading "Know thy partner," and strung on the neck-chain you never, ever take off, even in bed. Because if the voice you defer to and take to be your trusty superego belongs, instead, to your parents, friends, religious educators, or hometown social arbiters, where's the free will? If you, like me, find the received wisdom of your tribal elders to be *fundamentally* sound, on the core values, that is, then score a big win for us: Somebody did a proper job in rearing a good human being. But does that mean we must listen to *every*thing we were told? (If our moms had dutifully listened to their own puritanical moms, by my reckoning, a whole helluva lot of us—me, for one—wouldn't be here.)

Hard vs. Soft List

Think of your hard vs. soft list as a seesaw. The flip side of hard/no might be soft/maybe, meaning the seesaw can tip from hard into soft. That's why preset coded safe words and/or gestures are vital. We conclude this section with ideas for such words and gestures.

Safe Words and Gestures

If at any time in the exercise of DSRP you feel more than just a bit uneasy, if you're freaked out, feeling hurt (emotionally or physically), or repulsed, it's time to spring your scene-stopper safe word, letting your partner know to stop, *immediately*.

Here's the hard part: some girls (including this one) find the prospect of yelling "RED," "MERCY," or other off-the-rack safe word cheesy-embarrassing. The answer is to give some thought to coming up with a word or phrase that will do the trick without making you feel like a doofus. "NO! Mean it!" is a possibility. Uttered with the proper emphasis and in the right tone, it should damn well cue him that you're serious. Then, after a beat, a simple "Phew," and perhaps a short account of what rocked the boat and triggered alarm, should save embarrassment on both sides. Meaning, the two of you should feel free to resume the kinky, red-hot scene play.

If you're to be gagged, obviously you'll need to establish a safe gesture rather than a word, e.g., tossing your head from side to side, tapping him, making an insistent muffled *mmmmm* sound (accompanied by eyes in alarm-mode). Snapping your fingers is a good one, too. If you are gagged, he needs to know to be extra aware and alert to your body language, to be sure he "reads" your safe gesture.

More on safe words: Yes, they can be a scene spoiler, for the night or—let's hope not—forevermore, but I'm not going to hedge. Many handbooks I've seen promote safe words as reliably fail-safe firewalls, so, y'know, not to worry. Well, that's not always the case. *Do* worry. And *do* understand that successfully calling out your safe word in objection to something your partner is doing will stop the action. A bummer. But if you feel you *must* use your safe word, then use it and play be damned. When and if that happens, however, I suggest a salvage operation.

You just dropped your code-red word bomb, and everyone's rattled, feeling awkward and/or sheepish, the scene smashed into a million kinky pieces. Know that it's in your power to save the situation, if you wish.

Do not speak.

Tensions are understandably high and words will only compound the stress. Try to stay super-calm and to be reassuring.

Your having to resort to the safe word may have embarrassed him, made him feel abusive, guilty for causing you to call out "No," or inadequate and deflated as a lover who must have missed the how-to-be-smooth lesson. It happens.

You might try gestures that translate and convey to him, "Hey, I'm okay. It's okay. I'm not mad. Don't feel bad. Let's continue." Such gestures could include cocking your head down with a coquettish expression, playfully batting your eyes, smiling. Try to avoid a jerking up of the head, which is a common reaction to shock, as it will signal anger and imminent aggressive payback. (Uh-oh, I've done it now . . . *duck!)* Conversely, lowering the head is a signal of submission to most mammals. It says, "Don't want a fight, not gravely pissed off, in no mood for combat."

Next, initiate sexual or affectionate play with him. Lick his nipples. If your hands are free, rub his chest or penis, or stroke his arm.

If you are not gagged or are able to speak through your loose mouth gag, after calming him through body gestures, you might further reassure him and resurrect the spirit of play by coyly saying, " I want to suck your ****. I know I was a very bad girl for stopping you.

What do I have to do to avoid punishment?" Yes, yes, sounds belittling to you, but do remember that this is all play and, in the present context, "Sally was a bad girl" is fun role-play game-talk that can smooth over hurt feelings. Even when I've had to call out my safe word to a pro like Mr. H, I can tell he feels a bit mad at himself and guilty for "fucking up." So to speak, ahem.

Now, if you are fully tied up and gagged, and you've done your safe, head-tossing gesture, and he's put a halt to the action, then before the gag comes off, work your soothing body language. No frowny-face broadcasting, "You're screwed, babe!" Rather, I suggest first lowering your head to your chest or down to the side—an olive branch gesture. Start to spread your thighs and/or arch your back, exposing your lifted breasts to him. If hog-tied and mouth-gagged, rub your head against him or rub your head into the bed sheets. The idea here is to show playfulness through girly, sensual body gestures to quickly melt that frozen-in-memory scene-spoiler moment. It's up to you to show: no ice-out, everything's cool, let's continue, I'm okay and want to move on, let's get back into our play groove.

Then, once you've calmed the waters and resettled his jumpy nerves, he should be able to relax, ego intact, without feeling the need to get defensive.

Safe to proceed.

What if, however, you suspect that your guy has gone too far or pushed past your limits *on purpose*, without permission? Then you should *not* proceed. Stop the scene and either teach him a lesson then and there or simply break up with him! I'm serious. Very few men I know, and none of the men I like and respect, would purposely disregard their partner's limits. If it's not consensual, it's abuse. And that's all there is to that.

Whether you're dealing with a Good Guy or an Asshole, if developments have spoiled the mood for you, and you feel you just want to call it a night, you will still want to deal with the immediate situation *immediately*.

Smooth things over with Good Guy (WWSD? She herself may have said it best: "Tomorrow is another day"). Confront Asshole.

When dealing with Good Guy, who maybe just flubbed it: Pause for a bit as you compose yourself. Then calmly and nurturingly say, "It's not your fault, mistakes can happen in the frenzy of play." Or, "I didn't know my limit until we hit it, and now that we both know my threshold, this shouldn't, *cannot*, happen again." Give him a hug or some other show of affection to make him feel good, if you intend to stop the scene. The goal is to show that everything is back to normal. Ask him if he wants a glass of water, a cigarette, food. That will signal to him that you're trying to get past it, letting him know that he has nothing to worry about, even though you are shutting down scene play for the eve. Next time you play, you can remind him what happens when he gets carried away.

When dealing with Asshole who willfully skirted the rules: Best to pause for fifteen seconds, collect your wits, and calm yourself. If you don't, you'll likely get aggressive and feed into the SOB's sadistic delight in getting a thrill out of your pain and distress. If you want out and your lover is feeling "caught" but unrepentant, the calm approach is the safest in order to avoid raw-nerve fighting. If you read his actions as a momentary lapse in judgment and sense and are hearing feelings of remorse, that fifteen seconds of stonewalling silence will panic him and position you as strong and in control. Pretend you are scolding an unruly child (you are). Tell him you feel ambushed, are disappointed in him and his unforgivable behavior, that you are going to need space and time away from him before you can even consider moving forward. After all, he has broken an inviolable rule he agreed to play by, and you would be wise to ask that he leave immediately and wait to hear from you, after you have had time to think about whether you see fit to accept an apology. (If Asshole is a live-in partner who's circumstantially showing his true colors, uh-oh. Maybe time to rethink the arrangement?) Do *not* reward bad behavior by letting him "make it up to you" or by accepting his apology on the spot. Best to make him sweat a bit, as he comes to realize that you are not going to just give in, now or in the future. If you do take him back, let him work to regain your trust.

If you're sensibly looking out for number one, heeding the cautions in this guide, and being responsive to your own pop-up alerts (that early-warning system we smart and savvy chicks have cultivated since puberty), it's unlikely you will have to cope with too many men of the asshole class. I mean, they do sorta strut around with a scarlet *A*-for-*asshole* on their chests, no? (Yes!) Healthy men see sexually satisfying their partners as an irresistible challenge. It's a source of pride in a man who has his shit together that he is able to satisfy his lover, and he will remember what you liked and didn't like and try to impress. Sure, there are quickie-and-roll-over guys, but unless he's *your* guy, a partner in a stale relationship you're trying to resurrect, I doubt you're going to see him as the perfecto candidate for initiation into the high-stakes, high-payoff chambers of DSRP. You are proposing exciting hunter/captive role play that should stir lust for the hunt, the win, and the prize: domination of his lover, playfully, consensually, respectfully, in a dazzling realm that promises surprise, romance, and ecstasy. I suspect that even Snorie Bear can be turned into an energized Zorro.

My closing advice: Go slow. Stay sober.

INTERVIEW WITH MR. H

Mr. H ramps up the Big Talk on limits, now that you've broken the ice. Presented here as a Q&A between Alexis and Mr. H and offered as enlightenment into the guy's perspective.

Alexis: And now please address play limits from the male partner's point of view. Do men hate limits, resent them, feel constrained by or secure with them . . . what?

Mr. H: For men, knowing and *accepting* the limits is one of the most important things when it comes to bondage and role-playing scenes. For women, while it's good to expand boundaries and test limits, it's equally important to know exactly what you *can* and *cannot* handle. Initially, the drawing of limits may be uncomfortable for both parties, but the experience is doomed without them. Once you have touched on every possibility of your intended play, you need to sort things out: behaviors that you will allow, those that you are curious about allowing, and those that are completely off the table. It must be stated firmly, again and again, that hard limits are to be respected at all costs. Like the out-of-bounds lines on any playing field, guys need them!

Your soft limits, those that you are willing to push and explore slowly but surely, also count for a lot and should be discussed with your partner, who likely will enjoy the challenge of talking you out of (or into) them. Being gagged, for example, is one of the more controversial and angsty aspects of bondage, and if you say, "I'm curious but nervous about this," you free your partner to accept it as a soft limit. It will be a practice you approach slowly and carefully, using simple, comfortable methods to introduce and explore. Instead of a three-layer gag with stuffing, a ball gag and tape, you might open the proceedings with a cleave gag (a scarf pulled between the teeth, as used by the movie villain to keep the damsel in distress from screaming out her distress). The easy-does-it approach also is recommended with bondage and verbal play and certainly with any practice that involves aggressive physical interaction.

Getting back to your account of the *New York Observer* story on BDSM play among the Ivy League set, writer Rachel R. White reported these cautionary developments:

> *While the scene's mantra—"safe, sane and consensual"—is heard so often it might as well be translated into needlepoint, violations of these maxims are common. In the last year, hundreds of people have come forward to describe the abuse they've suffered within the scene. The victims are mostly women, and like 50* **Shades'** *fictional*

22-year-old Anastasia Steele, many are also young, submissive and uncertain about their boundaries.

You see, as White makes clear, why *no* must mean *no*. Hard limits, for men, are a test of respect and of self-control. Unlike the soft limit, which is an area of possible exploration and conversation, the hard limit is a big iron gate with a sign that reads DO NOT CROSS. A man who agrees to the limits and then proceeds to cross the line is not only disrespectful but also untrustworthy and dangerous. The rules of engagement begin with respect for yourself, and in abiding by those rules, your partner shows respect for them, and for you.

Alexis: Thanks. And amen.

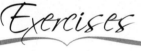

1. Break out your physical and mental lists of your brainstormed DSRP actions and words, those that turn you off and those that turn you on. Now we are going to amend the list. If the list includes items that have grabbed and continue to hold your attention, then move the "maybe" items to a "soft limit" column, even if you're on the fence about them.

2. Watch YouTube videos of children playing and of lions interacting. Pay attention to their body language and note how effectively their non-verbal signals convey intentions and express feelings. Consider what an impressive feat it is that these uninhibited, unconstrained beings are so successful in communicating their unambiguous messages through spontaneous gestures.

3. Place a chair in front of you. Imagine your lover sitting in it. Try something fun: Communicate to him what you want sexually, your safe sign and imagined reactions, through gestures and body language only. Aim for

spontaneity, living "in the moment." This will help open you up sexually, stimulate your creative imagination, and topple some of your socially conditioned defensive walls. With practice, you will awaken the femme fatale in you—your inner lioness—and free yourself from auto-adherence to the "bourgeois niceties" that stand in the way of passionate lovemaking. You're alone. Go for it. No one is watching.

4. Tell your partner (your real one, not the imaginary version!) an embarrassing secret. Alternatively, tell him five things you fear most; ask him to do the same. Then, with defenses down a bit, make love and introduce at least a smidge of DSRP. Maybe you convey that you're cool with his holding your hands down for a bit. Maybe you tell him, "I nibble you, and I agree to a light spanking." Get the show on the road.

The Promised Addendum: The Perils of Impromptu Play

An example of role play gone south due to lack of concrete communication between partners.

Good God, we've all had an awkward, I-wanna-pull-out-my-hair-and-run-into-traffic sexual experience with a guy. Ugh! C'mon, think back to that major yucky I-don't-wanna-think-about-it experience. Was it the first fumbling time you made out with a guy? Or the squandering your virginity story? Maybe that what-was-I-thinking one-night stand? Whatever. But, you know, the "big one."

I've dug painfully deep to tell you mine. *Sighs*. This was my cringe-inducing, just-erase-the-scene-with-bleach experience. A mess and not even worthy of being called a "hot mess," like a disheveled supermodel with hangover hair. So here we go.

Before my splash in the S&M scene, I was seriously dating a hot, sex god, playboy New York City rock star. He was into S&M role play but was by no means a connoisseur. He had "confessed" his S&M interests to me and cut to the chase. One late eve we plunged right on in. Bad, bad, bad. No preplay talks or discussion of my *yes, please*s and *no-no*s during play.

Scene 1: Alexis is tied up to a chair and left alone for forty-five minutes. Bam! This script lacks literary scene setting. Tied and waiting for what seemed like forever, my emotions went from a bit freaked out to furious and furiouser to sheer panic, accompanied by maddened sputtering like a raving nutter, on the order of "I'm gonna kill him! I'm. Going. To. KILL. Him! Mother F!"

When he finally came to retrieve me, I tried to stay calm and not ruin the night but I was visibly irate and lost it, demanding that he untie me, like *now!* He, too, was sputtering: "What? Huh? Sorry. I'm sorry. This always makes girls hot, turns 'em on." *Pfffffft! Well, not* this *girl, buddy* were my pissed-off thoughts, not verbalized but impossible to ignore.

All right, so his confusion and contrition did seem genuine, so let's give it another go, Alexis. He untied me but as if to compensate for his previous show of aloof remove, he began moving way too fast, way too hard. Rushing, taking a pass on any meaningful foreplay, retying my hands—forcefully, without finesse—gagging me quickly and tightly. "STOP!" I finally commanded. He did chill out, but I could see his neck vein popping in frenzied exasperation. Once again, he slowed down, trying to restore the romance of our rendezvous, but he was in such a nervous fluster that he jerked back into frantic play. "Wait! Can't you just hold up here!" said an infuriated Alexis. "Okay, I'm done, I can't do this with *you!*" he spit out as he jerked away in a frustrated, end-of-his-rope huff.

Scene 2: Alexis sits and pouts like a tossed-out hooker, untying herself and trying to regain some composure. Man storms off set, feeling like a first-class lout, flunking the audition for the Mickey Rourke role in the remake of *9½ Weeks*. Equally embarrassed, full of recriminations against each other, feeling dejected and like downright ass clowns, we didn't speak for a month. Epic sexual snafu. The worst!

The kink moral here is that it was neither his fault nor mine.

Simply, we were overreaching S&M newbies, victims of naïveté when it came to role-play protocols. If we'd established the rules of the road, at least talked shit out beforehand or drawn up a rough sketch, things wouldn't have gone so tragicomically awry. What did I learn here? That it's the submissive's responsibility to set the stage and sign off on the scene so that a partner's attempts at improvisation remain within her boundaries.

Okay, so I've finally talked it out, to you. I'm erasing it now from my short- and long-term memory. *Shiver, cringe, cringe.*

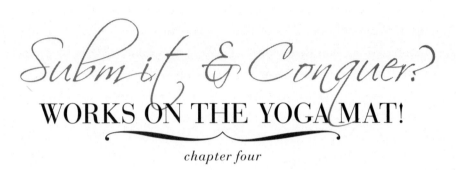

Submit & Conquer?
WORKS ON THE YOGA MAT!

chapter four

"So how long y'been practicing yoga?" I'm asked by a cute guy at the party. Not because I looked so damn fit or radiated peace and love, he laughed, but because he found the line a trusty icebreaker nowadays. What with yoga studios flourishing in cities and little burgs, in swanky gyms and suburban malls, and what with single chicks and cute house-wives answering the call of the ommmm, the guy was onto something. And he'd hit the mark with me.

I was a yoga girl for years before I was a "play" girl, and my first eureka moment in the DSRP world was: "This is *yoga!*" Here I am, sub-mitting to the discipline, shedding the self-centered mini-me to expose the Big Me, and entering that magical sub-space that I find calming and, paradoxically, stimulating. Through drama class exercises and yoga practice, I'd trained myself to recapture a feeling or mental state *at will* (similar to self-hypnosis, a handy, trainable skill). Which means that, when it came to sensual role play, I was *there* in no time, surrendering to the scene, to my partner, to the transporting ecstasy of "letting go." As an adolescent, I'd felt this same magic as I sat on the back of my horse, removing the bit and giving my mount his head, trusting him to give me an exhilarating ride and to bring us home safely (n.b., exercising horse sense is as important as developing man sense. He, Prussia, my first love, was a strong, intelligent, big-hearted beast of noble bearing, and the guy never let me down.)

What follows in this chapter is a gloss on the whole submission thing—explaining all I've learned about how submission can yield rewards. First, I offer a "dear diary" type story of how I "got over" the hump and learned to submit in DSRP, and second, I describe a revelation (my revelation) clarifying the mind-body equation that makes the self-indulgent act of submitting a singularly delightful discipline, not unlike what you might experience in yoga.

GROWING UP IN MANHATTAN, CHILDREN ARE passed protectively from hand to hand—from parent or nanny to friend's parent or nanny or to trustworthy doorman—which leaves only summer sleep-away camp for courting the bewitching dangers of independent capers. Such restraints left me chafing at the bit, singing, "Is this all there is?" and it wasn't until the summer between nursery school and kindergarten, when I began spending time with my country cousins, that I learned what I was missing: the liberty of roughhousing, away from the watchful eyes of caretakers. Life in the rural hinterlands of southern Indiana, and in the sand dunes on the shores of Lake Michigan up north, gave those lucky kids—and now *me!*—a *play* outlet. We skirmished as cops and robbers, cowboys and Indians—games in which feelings of aggression and fear were played out *hard*. We gave as good as we got, and then we'd put an end to the rowdy fun and games and . . . go have a Popsicle.

As adults, we don't have that kind of outlet (unless you count video games, a solo activity and a physical workout only for the thumbs), and I, for one, was sorry to be done with, to have outgrown, the mischief making. Having come to appreciate firsthand the concept of play as catharsis, and having seen how powerful feelings can be sweated out through freewheeling kids' play, I took to the delights of sensual role play hungrily and pronto. The knotty problem, for me, lay not in the exercise of kink but, rather, in my historical bugaboo: bowing to authority. Submission meant everything I constitutionally wasn't (and wasn't up to feigning): meek, compliant, humbly obedient, servile, and all the rest of those fawning fifties female words.

My conversion (to put a rapturously dramatic spin on it) passed through two introductory stages: the left-brain stage, in which I reasoned, analyzed, asked myself, "What's in it for me?"; and the right-brain stage, in which I got creative with it all, seized the metaphorical and experiential connections. All the world's a stage, no? Yes, it is. Do I not eagerly surrender my ego in the yoga studio and in the extreme sauna rooms? Yes, I do.

Then, on the threshold of taking the plunge, I quit dithering and faced myself. For readers on the brink, here's my to-plunge-or-not-to-plunge checklist:

Will the act of submission endanger my sense of self-worth, pride, self-respect?

If all the groveling, slobbering, bowing and scraping, and yessirring I pulled out for that state trooper at the radar trap on LA's I-5 didn't send me into self-esteem therapy, I figured, it wasn't likely I'd cave over a DSRP romp. 'Sides, it's back to power-neutral, my honeybunch, before the rooster toots reveille.

Must submission translate as weakness?

Lemme see, I thought to myself. I submit to all sorts of rules and regs and indignities every day. I stop at red lights, I step into the wind cage at the bidding of airport security, I scoop the kitty litter and bag the dog's curbside deposits—and so does my partner—and we don't feel weak or degraded. In any case, showing mutual respect for each other's rights across the board makes us both feminists, in my book.

In role-playing the submissive, am I endorsing or perpetuating the patriarchal status quo?

Easy one: no/maybe. To wit: Here's Dana Goldstein, a blogger for the *Nation,* a respected periodical self-described as "the flagship of the left." Citing a basic contention of sex-positive feminism, Goldstein suggests that "asking for what you want in bed is a feminist political act—whether you want to tie your partner up, be spanked by him/her or be tenderly made love to with lots of kissing."[1] In other words, it's the *asserting* of sexual preferences, not the choices themselves, that constitutes our modern declaration of independence and earns the feminist hallmark. Whereas our primitive, sexual instincts are old—really, *really* old—and are not ours to change (biologists fiddling with gene modification may get somewhere with that, but I hope not), it's the freedom to choose and to declare our penchants that's new and wonderful. Therefore, when considering whether I was ready to submit, I judged that, for a woman who will not be patronized or infantilized by her man or any other, I could afford to test the concept of "sweet surrender." That said, I acknowledge that I'm drawn to the masculine male who knows a battle-axe from a carving knife and is handy with both.

Does my appetite for DSRP make me abnormal?

Statistically, I realized, I had to accept that the "sex with a twist" that I fancy qualifies as "deviant," that is, different from what's considered average and generally acceptable, because polls show that a only small percentage of women pledge allegiance to aberrant sex (the numbers are low but trending upward). And I was fine with that; I felt no need to defend my personal code of conduct, and I didn't. More interesting to me were numbers from a study in the 1970s showing that up to 49 percent of women *fantasized* about submissive scenarios during sexual intercourse, with 14 percent doing so frequently.[2]

THERE CAME A POWER SURGE. I was *ready*.

> *Well c'mon*
> *Now I'm ready to close my eyes*
> *And now I'm ready to close my mind*
> *And now I'm ready to feel your hand*
> *And lose my heart on the burning sands*
> *And now I wanna be your dog*
> —"NOW I WANNA BE YOUR DOG,"
> IGGY AND THE STOOGES (1969)

So *that's* how this submission thing goes? Mr. Iggy Macho Animal Pop singing *our song*, inviting us to the sing-along, la la la la now I wanna be your *dog*? Reducing us to drooling lap puppies groveling in submission to our men? Fie! I say. Just *fie* on that yawny, has-been brush-off. Let those who will denounce DSRP as reinforcing demeaning sexual stereotypes. Whatever happened to "live and let live" (L&LL in Twitterspeak) anyway? As for me, DSRP casts a decided shadow, but where screeching Commissarinas and our tsk-tsking old-maid aunts see darkness, I see noir: mystery, sensuality, expectation, the fathomless Black Hole of Abandon. Irresistible.

For DSRP aficionados, submission in role play is the grown-up equivalent of "let's pretend." It is enlivened by a frisson of danger playing out through the imagination: I'm blindfolded or I'm tied up, *eeeee!* What's coming next? Playing by the rules, you and your partner have agreed to this power exchange, cast in complementary but unequal roles, and thus, your playmaster holds the cards, as you wish. It's within his power to make it a creative adventure, notwithstanding the naysayers who fear the art of enticement the way those Al-Qaeda troublemakers are said to fear the female body: OMG, it is too powerful, too seductive, we must place a force field over it, contain its voodoo! Ha!

No. Let's get it straight so we don't get it twisted.

People who look at consensual sexual submission with disdain, as a practice that's demeaning, degrading, or humiliating to women, have little understanding of what submission is and are seemingly unaware of its power-enhancement potential for women. Again, we're talking consensual, because if one does not submit to role play through the exercise of free will, that which unfolds is called taking, not giving. Submitting, then, becomes a sign of strength, in that it shows you to be secure in yourself and in your position within the relationship. It entails not identity correction but the willed suspension of certain personality traits—*for the duration of the "playdate."* DSRP can build greater self-awareness through exploration of this new state of being (surrendering) and thereby stimulate mental growth and strength.

And again, sexual submission is a gift you give yourself, not someone else, members of the Sourpuss Gladiatrix Corps be damned. Have those doctrinaire feminists, I wonder, browsed a copy of the latest (ninth) edition of *Our Bodies, Ourselves* and been surprised to see that the editors have included a section on DSRP? (I'd call it a tentative endorsement.) This is the resource the *New York Times* has called "America's best-selling book on all aspects of women's health" and a "feminist classic." And in a letter to the *New York Times*, the book's editors have answered a critic's nostalgia for earlier editions by saying, "With each new edition, *Our Bodies, Ourselves* evolves to stay relevant and accessible to its readers." Exactly so.

Rachel Kramer Bussel, the editor of the Best Sex Writing series as well as more than forty anthologies, calls feminist criticism of BDSM "misplaced." "The criticism that by default, female submission is anti-feminist, is insulting, infantilizing and condescending," she writes. "It conflates what happens in BDSM play under consensual and desired conditions with abuse, which is the opposite."

And from prima-iconoclast Camille Paglia: "I state in *Sexual Personae* that sex is a far darker power than feminism has admitted, and that its primitive urges have never been fully tamed: My theory is that whenever sexual freedom is sought or achieved, sadomasochism will not be far behind."[3]

I turn to these outside voices perhaps defensively, to counter the inner voices of misgiving that may begin to clamor in response to what I consider fusty and misguided critical attitudes. Coulda woulda shouda regrets are harder to face than a face-down with propriety. That's my precocious take on things, ventured well before the rocking-chair age when revisiting love and loss, the road not taken, is said to make strong wo/men weep. If submitting to the imposed patterns of social conditioning has you suppressing sexual needs, desires, or fantasies (even benign perversions), I brashly suggest: Better to be a let's-pretend slave to an amorous trusted partner than a slave to convention. Time to chuck the fears and worries and take back the keys to your own bedroom. Yes!

And here I yield the podium to the outspoken king of the irreverent put-down, acknowledging that I'm not the first to call on the late, great journalist H. L. Mencken in defense of contrarian opinion. Fittingly, his epigram (oft quoted in paraphrase, as here) is one of my faves: Puritanism is the haunting fear that someone, somewhere, is having a good time.

Bravo! Well done! And that's all I have to say about that.

FOR ME, BEING DEEPLY INTO A state of submission feels like being suspended in time. My senses are fully awakened but percolate underground. Submitting and surrendering, I pull free from negative sensory blocks, social conditioning, racing-slash-vexing brain tsunamis: unfinished business, pressing personal issues, and stresses. In surrendering my ego and my controlling instincts to another, I find myself introduced to myself, or, rather, that which I see as my guileless, artless "core self." I have learned in these moments to separate myself from my fragile, pesty ego, which, annoyingly, lives life vulnerable to inflation and deflation. The idea of exposing your true self, even to yourself, sans ego, might seem to be a nervous-making proposition, but if you're unflinching enough to let another wrest control, and assured enough to "lose yourself," it seems safe to wager you're going to like what you find. If not, fix it!

Who are we without our egos? We learn the answer when we lose control—or, more accurately, the illusion of control. By submitting and allowing another to guide us, we lock into the present (his control, his present) and are freed from our mucky brain blocks, from the past and future. Accepting a master, we master ourselves.

BELOW, I POSE A DEEP QUESTION that might be answered for you in the submissive state and provide some male feedback on the laws of attraction, gathered during a pop-anthropology "dig."

Who are you when you submit and yield control?

The "who" who "shows up" is a whole and authentic person, stripped of pretense, inhibitions, and defensive impulses. She's your personhood, distinct from your persona (from a Latin word for *mask*), which is the protective facade we present to the world to make the "right" impression on others. It's an artificial personality that's part real individuality and part answer to society's expectations. One cannot say that our personas don't serve a purpose—how many friends would we have without our gracious little white lies?—only that in stripping down to our core selves we can begin to contemplate our true nature and how we'd prefer to engage life. Ironically, DSRP can leverage our escape from the role-play vise our personas can become when we mistake them for our true nature and become nothing but a cultivated cover.

The Goddess Within

Because I was curious to know, and figured you might be as well, whether the submissive state is seen as weak, insipid, or unattractive (by men, natch), I decided to do a little intelligence gathering. In a self-selecting survey, over the course of a few months, I popped out my iPhone and showed to thirty or so men of varying age, social position, and political persuasion, images of two illustrious paintings depicting powerful females—one symbolic, one mythological—and asked for their snap judgment on the subjects' appeal. Without revealing my objective, I variously broached the inquiry in the context of interpreting body language, art history, even, in the age of implants, the aesthetics of breasts. In the course of an ostensibly aimless conversation, I'd sometimes ask which of the paintings they'd rather own or which of the women they'd prefer to (no, not bed/wed—a loaded question) know, anything to get them talking about the maidens.

The iconic works, admittedly and intentionally arch choices, were Delacroix's *Liberty Leading the People* and Botticelli's *The Birth of Venus*. Both women are barefoot and bare-chested, Liberty obliviously so, Venus, with arm brought across chest in a halfhearted nod to modesty. Liberty Gallic-handsome and brunette, Venus Renaissance-comely and strawberry blond. Neither looks undernourished.

Does it surprise that *not one* of my pollees expressed a preference, sexual or otherwise, for the valiant lady Liberty? Yeah, me neither. What was unforeseen was the uniformity of negative/positive comment vocabulary. Each of my free-associating respondents (all men I'd call "evolved" and none perceived as a misogynist) pejoratively applied the designation "feminist" in appraising Liberty, while qualifying their non-PC aspersions with various critical adjectives: sour, aggressive, crazy, mean, hostile, scary, troublemaker (out of the blue, the respondent who labeled her thus said, "I'd never hire her!"). Not one mentioned finding her physically attractive, although a couple joked sarcastically about her elevating the image of the French infantry.

Venus/Aphrodite was the runaway fave from every perspective, but, again, the comments were surprising—and intriguing. Since she is posed submissively, not aggressively, I'd thought it possible that some might find her aspect insipid, but none came close to that appraisal. The goddess of love and beauty is voluptuous, serene, *naked*, but most of the men's remarks on her sex appeal homed in on her beauty as essence rather than physical attribute. The adjectives they chose were: calm, serene, guileless, vulnerable, gentle, pure, innocent, and, yes, *feminine*. No one used the word *receptive*, but that was the message that came through, and it was clear to me that they were responding to her openness. A good word, *receptive*.

Now, both Liberty and Venus/Aphrodite are powerful women of passion and legendary strength. I, and I suspect most women, can relate favorably to both. Shown a picture of Teddy Roosevelt charging into war, would we let that define the man? Would we recall only the Rough Rider and not the statesman and avuncular good guy? So what's with the men and their single-minded focus on heroic Liberty's battle cry (*cri de guerre*, in the instance)?

I posed the question to a psychologist friend (female). She debunked my "science lite" survey—"wouldn't pass peer review," she laughed—but, playing along, she said, "It's the limbic system, darling!" To paraphrase her tossed-off comments, the limbic system controls feelings of pleasure related to our survival, e.g., eating, sex (that pretty much does it for the men, no?!). "So," I asked, "what was triggered in the brains of my subject males was likely in response to the goddess's unselfconscious sensuality? Her attitude of receptivity?" "Exactly." "So, it's all neuroscience?" "Pretty much," she giggled. "Your guys found Liberty alienating. They couldn't get past her assertiveness, her seeming lust for control, her dominance, not to mention the musket in her left hand! Not even her womanly curves and her beautiful full breasts communicated 'nurturance.'" Whereas, I thought, our goddess chooses not to wear her superpowers on her sleeve, so to speak, and wins the hearts and minds of modern mortal men by radiating openness and vulnerability.

So there you have it. I might have gotten the same answers from a Pygmy or a Marine or the metrosexual across the hall. Unfair but hardwired: Liberty works in the boardroom, but in the boudoir, not so much.

So how did I, more Liberty than Venus in bearing, learn to ease into and embrace the submissive play role? Admittedly, I'm kinda angry, kinda defensive, kinda insecure, kinda narcissistic, kinda aggressive. Well, maybe more than kinda. I dig in my heels in the face of authority and in the presence of swaggering, aggressive men. Kinda alpha bitch. I'm working on it. *Sighs.* I was birthed a full-blooded Aries hotty-totty with a pronounced case of penis envy. Heavy go-getter, stressed-out, confident, bossy mess hanging on by a string in this phallocentric world. My point? (Yeah, I talk too much, too. Add that to the list.) Not a naturally submissive woman. Dominant to the point that most men can't handle it and want to run. I prefer to pick up the dinner bill, don't accept extravagant presents, incessantly give/force my finger-waving opinions. Just how I roll. If a dutiful sales clerk IDs me for a cigarette purchase, I go into a rage. At parties and in bars, I'm compelled to confront and emasculate every slightly cocky guy. When my fetish film business employees (all males) f'd up or slacked off, I'd throw fits and objects, my face contorting into that of a tyrant-ugly monsteress. Not attractive or healthy, eh? Nope.

Submitting sexually and playing with DSRP both repelled me and saved my life—well, that may be a stretch, but def my well-being. Similarly, yoga had helped to calm my high-voltage go-go-go intensity and domineering personality, but, as far as curing me of my churning penis-envy anger issues, yoga was, to invoke the old trope, like bringing a knife to a gunfight.

My first experience with a knock-out submission similar to that of DSRP was in the sauna at my health club. The hotter the better. I'd lie naked in body bag form on the bamboo boards and suffer the heat for up to an hour, watching as other (sensible) girls scurried out in less than half that time. As the minutes ticked away, I surrendered fully to my master—the heat. I felt half conscious, pleasantly aware that Master Heat had broken me. With my natural defenses on lockdown in hibernation mode, all the pent-up anger, stress, and frustrations therapeutically sweated out into the bamboo floorboards. Those hardwood slats might have been paddles, so effectively did they co-conspire with the brutal heat to pummel me into submission.

Post sauna-workout, a jump on the 6 train to yoga class. I noticed that in my serene submissive state, people would smile at me, men would flash me way more sexual looks, and people would kindly excuse my inadvertent body slams as the subway lurched around curves and bounced me around like a pinball. Suddenly, life was a calm walk in the park. I floated to yoga class and explored bizarre animalistic pretzel origami stretches. By the next day I was . . . back to bitch. FuckUghArrrgh!

One of my simpatico girlfriends, an alpha businesswoman and fellow monsteress slitting throats during the workday, suggested I read a blog she'd discovered, *H Is for the Hunter*. She said she'd been giving BDSM a try, as the submissive, in role play with her boyfriend, and that it had improved their relationship and toned down her cat-on-a-hot-tin-roof-bitch-witch-from-hell state. I took a skeptical peek and found Mr. H's explicit and detailed scenes of his sexual domination of women. A secret turn-on, but my blockage said, "No! C'mon, I'm not some freaky-kinky girl. I dig the good ol' sweaty mission-style sex." I had a deep-seated phobia of being restrained—in *any* situation—and this seemed strange, cracked-up bizarre-o-ness.

You'll read the story of how I met the charismatic blogger Mr. H in chapter 7. When I did, I submitted, surrendered, was restrained, a bit humiliated, commanded, controlled—and, reflexively, I fought back. Then I shut out Alexis and her monsteress ego, and, wow! I enjoyed it. Just wow! Well, slap my arse and call me Sally, there's hope for Miss Priss! Alexis became a sub girl for the night and felt a release of body, mind, and ego that was unlike any I'd ever experienced through any practice or health regimen. And! The effects lasted longer than a night, longer than a chill pill. A week, at least. The sexual role play forced me to confront my worst fears, anxieties, and pride (verging on hubris) issues. In weekly dose after weekly dose, I explored, I grew, I changed. I let go of controlling phobias (e.g., being restrained), and in surrendering to them I became cool, calm, collected, balanced. In role play your thoughts are directed, your cares banished, by another. You get to just *be*, soaking up all sensations, as if someone is serving you. Becoming zero can release you from ego jail, that clamorous knocking on your brain that drives you to a weak, stressed state that dictates, "*Go! Succeed! Control!*" Relentlessly. So where's the balance? DRSP gives you that. You can't beat that with a stick, whip, yep.

Submission in DSRP: Forbidden Territory?

I was awfully curious to see what very observant people of some of the popular world religions thought of BDSM. I conducted endless Google searches for answers to the question, "Is BDSM allowed in [fill in a religion]?" and perused hundreds of responses from religious followers, some towering figures in their communities, citing scripture from the various holy books. What I discovered, first off, was that all the popular forums of every major religion entertained, in some form, the basic question: "Is BDSM allowed?" Surprisingly, by my estimate, about 90 percent of the commenters on the various religious forums ventured that it *was* permissible, with some exceptions and within certain parameters.

Every religious message board seemed to offer scripture in support of the essential message that as long as there is mutual consent and no "harm to the body," DSRP practice is condoned within marital sex. DSRP is allowed if it is done with care and consent and with the intention of bringing the couple closer together. The few naysayers who repudiated the arguments of the commenters, arguing that such behavior is forbidden by their region, referred predominantly to sadist and masochist practices, which, I agree, are unhealthy and abusive. Sadists need or wish to inflict pain, and they do so with or without consent. Masochists are pain-hungry/obsessed and don't sweat the "consents." DSRP is not S&M. Or, more correctly, DSRP players are not necessarily BDSM players. Just as the moderate social drinker does not deserve automatic inclusion in the Drunks' Club. I do not condone the extreme practices of BDSM play, in this book or otherwise. This guide is intended for the light to medium drinker, to extend the metaphor.

Yoga and DRSP Submission

When one is in a DSRP state of submission, she is practicing yoga. What?! 'Tis true. Non-yoga practitioners may be muttering comments such as I heard from a friend via Facebook:

> *Isn't yoga for hippie-dip people who eat only room-temperature turnips and drink warm water and seem too lethargic to ever have sex? And if they do, you suspect that the guys can muster only a mooshy-gooshy half boner?*
> —(PREFERS TO REMAIN) ANONYMOUS

Uhhh . . . no, smart aleck.

Yoga works! Yoga has benefitted millions of people for thousands of years. Yoga is a five-thousand-year-old practice that in the past several decades has been embraced by the Western world, as can be seen by the proliferation of yoga schools, classes, videos, and magazines. Yoga is a scientifically proven stress reliever and delivers a unique meditative experience some people call "bliss."

One of the ancient definitions reads: "Yoga is the ability to direct the mind exclusively toward an object and sustain that direction without any distractions." So wrote Patañjali, the compiler of the Yoga Sūtras, an important collection of aphorisms on yoga practice, *two thousand years ago.*

Writes T. K. V. Desikachar, the son of Sri Tirumalai Krishnamacharya, who was known as the father of modern yoga: "That 'object' can be something concrete like a work of art, as dynamic as a runner's race."[4]

Extrapolating from that definition, does it not then follow that "that 'object'" can as well be a lover? I certainly believe so and further assert that the given activity can be DSRP. Like the yoga postures known as asanas, DSRP is a tool employed to dispel tensions and get the submissive into a full-concentration merge with an object—"the lover"—as DSRP transports the submissive to a humbled state, temporarily suspending the ego and liberating the mind from fears, inhibiting perceptions, and the obsessive drive to control.

The purpose of the asanas is to calm the body for meditation, allowing the practitioner to develop a "lucid, balanced mind in our distracting, stressful, and difficult societies," and, ultimately, "to bring Man into contact with something beyond himself, and far greater."[5]

Some yogis dismiss the idea that DSRP, like yoga, can bring a submissive to a meditative state, but I believe that Krishnamacharya would not have been among them. Even though his teachings were deeply rooted in the yoga scriptures, his expression of Patañjali's yoga was decidedly secular, as reflected in this instruction to a class, recalled and reported by a former pupil: while leading a meditation, Krishnamacharya asked students to close their eyes and "think of God. If not God, the sun. If not the sun, your parents."[6]

Krishnamacharya, an ayurvedic (i.e., a system of traditional medicine native to the Indian subcontinent) healer and scholar, practiced and taught yoga as a means to sustain and restore health and well-being—physical, mental, and spiritual—to those he treated, but, as his "God-sun-parents" directive reveals, he did not "preach" yoga as a religion. As a matter of fact, at the closing ceremony of the Yoga into the 21st Century conference in New York City, in September of 2000, his son offered these comments on the subject of the relationship between hatha yoga and religion: "Yoga was rejected by Hinduism because yoga would not insist that God exists. It didn't say there was no God but just wouldn't insist there was."[7]

Too, as a result of the teachings Desikachar received from his father and other instructors, he approached every student as "absolutely unique," in the belief that the most important aspect of teaching yoga was that "the path of yoga means different things for different people"[8] and, therefore, that each person should be taught in a manner that he or she understands.

Such is the philosophy of the large-minded yoga instructors (all of whom call themselves teachers, not yogis) I have always sought out. One of them, in response to my question as to whether a DSRP lover could qualify as an "object" of yogic focus, answered, "Why not?"

Objectification

Objectification is a fairly extreme submissive action in DRSP, and it can lead to a soothing, meditative state.

Objectification is a DSRP scenario in which the sub acts as an inanimate object, remaining completely still, immobile. For example, a dominant may instruct a sub to be a "table," or simply not to move. Subs describe the objectification experience as bringing on a trance-like state. As in meditation, the point is to dispatch distractions, to remain absolutely still—have an itch? Don't scratch it—so as not to disturb the harmony of the mind-body connection. If the body moves, the mind follows. It is important not to break the trance in fixating on the object of *your* focus, that is, the dominant. At the same time, of course, immobilization of the sub is a means for the dominant to create illusionary absolute control over the sub. It fuels the heat.

To return to the teachings of Krishnamacharya, one finds meditation similarly described: "It is as if the individual has lost his own identity and achieved complete integration with the object of understanding."[9]

It's not that the object, in this case your dominant lover, is God or godlike, or even deserving of worship, but, rather, a conduit to something beyond yourself, a higher power, an inspiration. "For Krishnamacharya, [the phrase] 'surrender to yoga' meant directing all one's will toward achieving independence, an autonomy of mind and spirit."[10]

So, you see, ideally, your surrender to "that object," to your lover, is an act bigger than either of you.

Sub-Space Meditation: The Kind Version of S&M

Sub-space is a deep meditative state commonly reached through DSRP wherein the submissive feels relaxed, at peace, and in a sleeplike state. It yields incredible feelings of warmth and tranquility.

For our purposes, there are three important stages—called "limbs" in the ancient text—to mastering the state of meditation, each building on the next (I draw from the Yoga Sūtras of Patañjali). They may be defined as follows: *Dharana* is the direction of the mind toward a chosen object, which may be seen sensually by the practitioner; *Dhyana* is a state in which all mental activities form an uninterrupted flow only in relation to that object; *Samadhi* is the final stage ("Nirvana") when the subject's mind is merged with the object. "In Samadhi our personal identity—name, profession, family history, bank account, and so forth—completely disappears . . . nothing separates us from the object of our choice; instead we blend and become one with it."[11]

Through submission to a partner, the sub often experiences the aforementioned loss of ego and identity, in fully concentrating on, and in *counting on*, her dominant's guidance to free her overactive brain. The submissive enters a meditative state. The DRSP tools used to effect a meditative state may be foreign to most yoga practitioners but they're not against the "rules" of yoga, as the tools are employed in the consensual execution of sensual, erotic, and natural vehicles. Actually, I find being restrained and bound more challenging than the yoga postures. In bondage, the body is bound and restricted but the mind is set free. One learns to cast off anxieties, fears, and even slight discomfort by submitting to the physical restrictions, just as, in yoga, one assumes fixed positions and, with practice, overrides the body's initial resistance to achieve a deeper freedom.

IN CONSIDERING THE CONNECTIONS BETWEEN YOGA and DSRP, I was struck by the way an acquaintance of mine—a high-powered female attorney in New York City—described her attraction to DSRP (as a sub). In an email, she told me:

Being dommed is particularly intriguing to those who are "powerful"
in their own lives. It's a means to get away from the trials and
worries of one's "normal life" where one is in control most of the time.
When the person gives themselves over to the dom, there is a thrill
and anticipation of not knowing what will come next . . . but knowing
it will be pleasurable in some manner or form.

THE ATTORNEY'S SENTIMENTS WERE ECHOED IN an online, off-the-cuff conversation I had with a submissive DRSP player friend (who informed much of my research for this book). She: a writer, late forties, Yale graduate, has never taken a yoga class or meditated and knows very little about either practice.

After reading the unscripted discussion, you may decide for yourself if you think "sub-space" qualifies as a meditative state. In the spirit of the late Krishnamacharya (who died in 1989 at age one hundred), I'll try to allow you to come to your own decision—and I won't call myself a DRSP guru. Ha. We are not currently engaging in DSRP, so here you must assert your identity and opinion and retain the freedom to judge for yourself. Trust your gut. If this sounds right to you, it is. You are the master here.

Alexis: Anywaay . . . I was going to go back to your wonderful email describing sub-space. Can you describe it further?

Mary (pseudonym): I think the best description is like being in a zero-gravity zone. All the baggage of your mind is lifted and you float around the room. It is a mix of a physical feeling—relaxation and lightness, a floating sensation—with an emotional feeling—warmth and well-being.

Alexis: What gets you there?

Mary: I find it comes from a sort of "crack." The dom pushes you to a place—and you could achieve this through a lot of means—where the sub would either crack up, fall into a heap in tears, or . . . push through to this place. I guess sort of like muscle failure if you were lifting a weight? You do another rep, another, another, till you just . . . cause a tear.

Alexis: You said it felt like "floating." Any other descriptions?

Mary: The overwhelming feeling is of lightness. Freedom from harm. A bit like being a ghost. Ghosts can fly around their enemies, they can wave their swords, but they can't do anything because . . . they're ghosts. It feels like that. You've switched over to this bodiless place where no one can harm you.

When I was a kid, the pastor told me, "Heaven is the feeling of being with God." That's what this is like also. The dom is your god and you feel you are now soul-bonded, very much the way (I imagine) in Christianity you are supposed to feel when you die and go to heaven: You feel the presence of God like an invisible arm wrapped around you.

The thing I think you might want to emphasize in the book is that the feeling of sub-space definitely has to do with all the issues and burdens of life falling away. Finally arriving at that space where all those anxieties and painful thoughts just effortlessly melt away and you are left with bliss. Very much like meditation, and I think you could make the case that it is a form of meditation.

P.S. I assume this experience is pretty much the same for people into very corporal things, canings and so forth . . . but I prefer light BDSM. I'm not into any physical pain. You arrive at a breakthrough point and feel this sensation . . .

Alexis: Would you agree it feels like your brain is "off" and you are present but not distracted by your surroundings?

Mary: I have always liked your "brain off" idea. I think it is *on* in the sense that you are hyperaware of the dom and of the scene. Very sensually aware of the feeling, the smell, the sound. But all the other stuff, the chatter of the brain, definitely *off*. It is really the "in the moment" thing everyone talks about. I think because it is so emotionally and sexually charged, it's easier to be in *that* moment than it is to focus on a mantra or a picture of a beach.

Alexis: Great! That "ghost" you mentioned would say that is you being introduced, so to speak, to your "true self," beyond your conditioning and misapprehensions. Your "true self" is not your ego; it's your core being, with its needs met and immune to harm. It is peaceful, untouched, and untouchable. Anyway, this is the place mediation should lead us to . . . and sadly most yoga practitioners think that traditional lotus-position meditation is the only way. In *The Heart of Yoga,* the guru Desikachar (though in fact he says he refuses to be called a guru or a yogi) says one can achieve mediation bliss by many means. Sub-space *is* a strong meditation. I'm going to try my best to get it on the map and seen that way.

Mary: That is a great image, that meeting of selves . . . where did you get it?

Alexis: I made it up . . . trying to explain it to you . . . meditation.

Mary: Perfect. There is an old Indian saying: "There are many ways to the top of a mountain."

I'll conclude the chapter with a horror story—a nightmarish account of sexual starvation (my own, and my fault!), before sending you off with a more uplifting set of yoga-pose exercises.

A Horror Story: No Time for S-E-X

In 2012, more women than ever are kicking ass in the workplace (yay!), racking up success stories (double yay!), and, sadly, paying the price. It's called $-T-R-E-$-$. If you're one of the trailblazing many, you've likely discovered, with dismay, that you're living your career in your head, at the expense of your body, and that you're drained, stressed to the max. Americans have come to accept this as normal—it's *not!*

This body-mind disconnect causes problems across the board but is particularly irksome when it manifests in the bedroom. How's your sex life these days, anyway? If the answer is, "Oh, nothing a few drinks after work can't fix," then you've already realized that alcohol is a quick fix at best. Works every time as an instant relaxer but, overall, it's not a healthy choice, unless you're into developing a desensitizing numbness over time. What most of us really crave is satisfying sexual relations . . . getting the red blood flowing, awakening the libido, and keeping it awake for longer than the, uh, quickie encounter.

When I was running my film business, and had employees to feed, I suffered Godzilla-size stresses. Responsibilities piled up, heaps upon heaps upon heaps of them, devaluating my sex life from wonderfully alive to D-E-A-D, for a very long time. To the point that it freaked out my psychologist! Referring to my then nonexistent sex life with a lusty, red-blooded boyfriend, she said, "This is a very, very bad sign and unhealthy." I was so-o-o-o in my head that I would shoo him away every time he wanted to get going. I was saying things I never thought I'd hear come out of my mouth: "I'm too stressed out." "I have way too much to deal with right now. . . no time!" Or, more often: "Not right now, *damn it!*" It got so bad that I once nastily snapped at him, in the off-putting voice of the deranged exorcist girl: "Why don't you go find someone else to sleep with! Just don't tell me about it!" And yes, I meant it.

Good God, I was seriously stressed and f'd up, obsessed with my business to the exclusion of all other areas of my life. The truth is, if I'd taken just one hour at night to sexually release with my partner, my business wouldn't have suffered, but I was suffering plenty. I was so tightly wound that even alcohol no longer had the power to loosen me up. I'd end up tipsy, still obsessed with business problems, and focused on the next day's agenda.

Then, a solution! Thank God! I finally forced myself to sneak off to the promise of a de-stressing yoga class. And it did the trick! After a yoga workout, with those heaven-sent body-stretching poses, I started to welcome nightly bed romp invitations from my partner. I'd regained a healthy, distanced perspective about work and life and became physically and emotionally relaxed enough to look forward to engaging in sexual activities, to the simple pleasure of being touched.

Resuming yoga practice led to the restoration of a healthy sex life (and later, great kinky role play) with my boyfriend. I'd forgotten how beneficial it could be. In fact, it was divine and just what I needed. But how, with epic stress levels, did I get myself into an adrenaline-reduced state, stripped of defenses, enough to be able to submit sexually to my partner? All credit is due the power of a five-thousand-year-old mental, physical, and spiritual discipline. Like watching ink suffuse through a whirlpool, I felt the amazing results of yoga in body and mind.

In my early twenties, I'd been yoga-obsessed, practicing four hours a day. I took an advanced yoga/meditation teacher-training course and earned the teacher certification. When I opened my film business, I felt I had no time for anything else—yoga or kinky play, which, as you read in this chapter, can put one in the same desirable mental place. Yoga and submissive role play can bring the same results, and, in fact, can be mutually beneficial (more on that topic later).

Whereas, during my stress marathon, I'd been popping anti-anxiety pills, like almost everyone else I knew, three months after resuming yoga practice and kinky role play, the anxiety pills began to leave me exhausted. My doctor explained that, as I now was relieving my adrenalin high through healthy activities, the medication was overkill.

The golden lesson of yoga is that mind and body are one. When one is sick or has suffered an injury, depression can easily set in. Physically relaxing the body through yoga's tension-relieving stretching and breathing techniques is curative, forcing the mind and body to open up. These poses force this opening up and, for women, the release of tension from the pelvic region. They help to compel the mind to follow the body, open up to new perspectives, and release mental compression. By extension, they help to open one mentally and physically to the joys and therapeutic benefits, physical and mental, of sexual role play. It's a very simple equation: Release the body from stress and you feel relief—and submission—all over. Yoga is a magic wand.

Physiologically, as both yogis and marathon runners know, pushing physical limits and working through pain results in the release of endorphins. S&M practitioners know it, too.

The yogi who led my teacher-training course explained that the most valuable poses are those that involve stretching the pelvis. As he explained it, the pelvis is the cornerstone of the body. The center point, it bears the heavy task of supporting the weight of the upper body and is the bowl that keeps the upper and lower body in balance. It is the part of the body that holds the most tension and supports the organs, muscles, and nerve grid. No surprise, then, that releasing tension from the pelvic region and sexual organs is nature's answer to relieving stress.

For the highly stressed, overworked woman looking to enhance the role-play experience, I offer eight easy-to-manage yoga poses selected from hundreds of such stretching/relaxing poses. I've chosen them for their power to ease tension in the pelvic region, as well as their ability to relax the body overall. There's bound to be at least one that delivers for you, so simply stick to those you like best and you'll feel the results.

Before we jump in, just a few suggestions intended for those readers who have not previously practiced yoga. If you find your thoughts racing and you can't turn your mind away from what you're going to make for dinner or the million things you have to do the next day, my advice is to quit trying to force your thoughts away, as that will only build more tension. Let them stay, but gently pass them through and out of your mind. Envision a paradise, a Caribbean beach, perhaps with dolphins at play. Or recall a time when you felt euphoric or simply at peace, maybe during a massage in a lovely spa. Again, if stressful thoughts intrude, don't fight them. In yoga, as in the submissive state of DSRP, a calm and uncontaminated state is achieved by overriding racing thoughts. In surrendering your mind and body, breaking loose from the enervating stress of maintaining self-control, you deliver yourself to the promised land of sensual role play, welcoming surprise and release.

As you progress from gentle to more strenuous stretching poses, try to follow the instructions but feel free to make adjustments to suit your comfort level; there's no my-way-or-the-highway authoritarianism about yoga poses. Many instructors—yours perhaps—would disagree, but I've learned to steer clear of the totalitarian yogis. My own wise yogi guru taught me to reject the idea of a single, one-size-fits-all model of body alignment associated with any yoga pose, as each body type is unique. To insist that yoga can be done only one way would be the same as saying that the only way to reach orgasm is by practicing the missionary position.

One last note: Yoga practitioners and instructors acknowledge the fifty shades possible in the coloration of a posture, through use of varying mental visualizations. Try mine! I think you'll rouse sexier and more sensual sensations following these interpretations. *Wink.

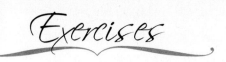

Exercises

First, eight yoga pose exercises:

1. *The Hot Bath Pose:* Think luxuriating soak in a sumptuous tub at a Palm Springs spa. Such is the voluptuous effect of this pose. Begin by sitting on the floor next to a wall and swinging your legs up so that your feet rest, with your legs slightly bent, against the wall, as you lower your back onto the floor; imagine you're submerging into a steamy bubble bath. You will end up lying perpendicular to the wall. You can place a fluffy pillow under your back or hips to make the pose more comfortable, and you might experiment with moving your hips closer to the wall or farther away, depending on the flexibility of your legs. You can let your arms rest at your sides, palms open to the sky, or bring them up over your head to achieve a side-body stretch. Place an eye mask or rolled-up towel over your eyes and just relax and feel the moment. The minimum time for results is fifteen minutes, though the longer you stay in the pose, the more relaxed you will feel. As your legs are above your torso, your blood flow is reversed, and when that happens, the "baroreceptor" arteries located on the sides of your neck immediately start to slow down your pulse rate and heartbeat. (BTW, the reason anti-anxiety pills are effective is because they induce the same physiological reaction.) The essence of this pose is to "do" *nothing.* Lie back and settle into the warmth of the room, channeling the comfort and security of hot bath water enveloping your naked body.

2. *The After-Orgasm Pose:* Lie down on the floor on your back with your arms comfortably at your sides, palms facing up. Bend your legs and scoot your feet approximately one foot below your buttocks. Place either a yoga block (purchased at any yoga school or online) or two or three hardback books, no more than eight inches high and covered with a towel, underneath the buttocks. The block/books should touch your

sacrum, the bone between your buttocks, but do not let it extend to your lower spine. Adjust the block/books to where you feel comfortable, then gently let your knees and legs fall to the sides with the soles of your feet of the floor. This feels soooo good. While your pelvis is in suspension, supported by the object, it has no weight to bear and thus can open and relax. Again, to enhance the experience, place an eye mask or folded towel or scarf over your eyes and enjoy. Hold the pose for ten minutes or longer. I could be in this pose all day. It feels that good.

3. *The Blossom Pose:* Get a couple of pillows or a bunch of rolled-up towels. Sit in an upright, cross-legged position on the floor. Place the pillows or towels underneath your knees. Then carefully stretch out your legs, placing the soles of your feet together. Then let the soles of your feet spread a bit apart from each other. Peel open your two feet, as if they are opening flower blossoms. Then, starting from your lower spine, try to bend over your feet, vertebra by vertebra, the slower the better. You may reach your hands and arms in front of you or place the hands on the tops of your feet (Posh Girl's choice). *Stop* bending over if you start to feel pain. A little discomfort is okay, as your body will adjust and relax as you stay in the pose. Close your eyes and feel the pelvis spread like a blossoming flower, the blood rushing through your entire pelvic region to wash away tension and awaken your sexual organs.

4. *The Elegant Armchair Pose:* Find a comfortable chair. This pose can be done at your workplace or on an airplane, wherever you can sit in a chair. Place your feet at hip distance or farther apart, whatever feels best (I like more than hip-distance apart), with the soles of the feet planted firmly on the ground. Again, starting at your lower spine, fold yourself over your legs slowly, vertebra by vertebra, drip by drip, like a gentle, cascading waterfall, until your hands are planted on the floor. (If your hands cannot easily reach the floor, it's okay to let them hang.) Hang like a rag doll. I like to shake my head "no," then shake it "yes" to loosen my neck. Then let your head hang like a ripened piece of fruit

about to fall from a tropical tree. Feel your pelvic and vaginal region sumptuously spreading apart and relaxing. Imagine the tropical sun kissing your body as you spread out and soak in the warm blood flow awakening your entire pelvic area.

5. *Café in Paris Pose:* This is more of a spinal twist, but now that we have relaxed the pelvis, it's time to raise the temperature and release the hard, cold, condensed pressure of the tensed spine weighing down on the pelvis. Lie on the floor. Imagine you're wearing that cute little dress you saw in the fashion magazine with glam sunglasses and you are sitting at your favorite Parisian café, feeling the breeze. Stretch out your legs and cross your right knee over your left in sexy, Parisian-café fashion. Then, keeping your torso and head flat on the ground, bring your café-in-Paris legs to your left and try to touch the floor with your right knee. Gently reach your left arm over to your right side, keeping your buttocks on the ground and your right arm above your head. Feel the silky release of your lower back and the twist of your spine as it lets go of all the tension and compression between your vertebrae. To go deeper, stretch and reach out your right arm and hand as far as possible, as if you are trying to grab the sexy little dress before it's snatched by the shopper mob. The more you reach, the more red Bordeaux blood will smooth out all the tight nerves in your spine. Ahhh . . . then repeat with the left knee over the right and the right arm reaching to the left. R-E-L-A-X.

6. *Swan Pose:* Imagine a majestic white swan with its pure white plumage puffing its curvaceous chest out while it floats in a sapphire pond. This is the essence of the Swan Pose: floating and divine. Begin by sitting cross-legged on the floor. Keep your right knee and leg bent and spin your left leg behind you, fully stretched out. Place a pillow or rolled-up towels under your right buttock to support your upright torso. Bring your shoulder blades back to kiss. Watch that your shoulders go back and down rather than hike up toward your ears. Open your chest like that of the beautiful curved and radiant swan floating on the smooth

water. Let your arms be your wings and elegantly wave them open to your sides. Take a deep breath in through your nose, and as you exhale through your mouth, gracefully bend over your right knee as far as you can. You can use pillows to support your upper arms or, if you are flexible, let your arms reach out in front of you. Then repeat with your left knee bent and your right leg stretched out behind and a pillow supporting your left buttock. This is the best hip and pelvis opener for non-super-advanced yoga practitioners, as it deeply opens your hips and pelvis while your body is relaxed and not straining. You may nestle into a deeper pelvic and hip opener by removing the pillow. Settle into the pose for five to fifteen minutes per side. The longer you hold the pose, the more fully you achieve the desired results, naturally.

7. *Lover's Pose:* This pose can be done alone or, greatly enhanced, with a lover. It's very simple. Sit on the floor with your legs stretched out in front of you, just inches apart. Your feet can be erect or fall to the sides. Place your hand underneath your right buttock and pull the flesh out from under you and back, away from your legs, then repeat on the left side. You will feel that this action spreads your vaginal and pelvic area so that you can stretch deeper. Now reach your arms up to the sky for a big relaxing stretch. Hold. In this stretch position you will notice that your lower back is not curved or slumped and your whole back is straight. Keep this posture. Take a deep breath in through your nose and as you release through your mouth, bend your torso forward from your lower back, stretching your arms and hands toward your toes. Try to touch your toes with your fingers. If you can't, no worries. The idea is to bend as far as possible forward and down, hinged at your lower back, with your arms and fingers extended. Imagine a bolt of warm light shooting from your lower back through your arms, out through your fingertips. Or you can imagine a lover massaging your back, placing his hand at the base of your spine and kneading up and up your spine to your neck, then gently pulling your arms in front of you, releasing them from their cramped shoulder sockets.

Now, it would be best if your lover could *actually do* this. How can you enhance this pose with a lover so that it feels orgasmic? Ask your lover to do a bizarre but OMG-does-it-feel-good action. While you are in the full, bent-over pose, have him simply lay his stomach on your lower-to-mid back area, his arms on the floor beside you for support. He then is to press his weight into your lower and mid back, while he takes deep belly breaths. Each deep breath you feel from his belly should press your belly farther into your legs, spreading your pelvis and tensed vaginal area. This is a common adjustment exercise in yoga, teacher to student. A yoga teacher did this to me in class, and the effect was as rousing and tension-relieving as an orgasm. Who says yoga doesn't get kinky? No wonder so many chicks are into it, huh? (Note: I've seen more painful pulling, pushing, and twisting from yogis pretzeling themselves into extreme positions than I ever saw from domme action on the most diehard masochists at the S&M dungeon. Each to her/his own maso-ritual, I always say! *Wink.*)

8. *Full Submission Pose:* After the previous seven poses, you now should be in a much more opened, relaxed, and receptive state of body and mind, ready to embrace giving in, letting go, submitting, and surrendering. In this last pose, just *be*, don't *think* or *do*. As if you were gently but firmly held in place, tied up to the bedpost of Scarlett O'Hara's puffy, romantic bed with silk scarves gently masking your eyes, your tethered arms and legs apart, feeling the support from the bed and your lover massaging your shoulders—that's the visual essence of this pose. You can relax, in full surrender, giving up all control and submitting to the lovely abyss of complete serenity.

Lie down on the floor on your back, legs stretched out, comfortable with a pillow under each knee and an eye mask or rolled-up towel over your eyes. Take your hand and pull each shoulder blade down your back to relieve shoulder tension. Then rest your arms comfortably by your sides with your palms facing up. Your job is to *do nothing*. They say this is the hardest pose in yoga, and therefore it's the pose that ends many yoga classes. It is hard not to move, to submit, to relinquish control and do nothing, but you must try to think of nothing, to become nothing, to reach the point where your stress, your pestering thoughts, and your muscle urges are turned off and you simply float. This is the ultimate state of relaxation, akin to submitting and surrendering control to your male partner in DSRP. The Sanskrit word *yoga* stems from the Sanskrit root *yuj*, meaning to control, to yoke, or to unite, and any time you lose your ego, lose yourself, give in to nothingness, and focus your surrendered thoughts on an object or person, you are connecting yourself like a yoke to something or to someone, and you are practicing the essence of advanced yoga. So yes, by completely submitting to your partner in DSRP, by losing yourself to a higher state of consciousness, you are engaging in a five-thousand-year-old restorative practice called . . . yoga. The poses are merely a way to get you there, to move you to that advanced state of surrender. Submit and enjoy!

*Now, three **DSRP** readiness exercises:*

1. Try to do at least one of the yoga poses and/or take a yoga class. It will ease you into exploring and experimenting with practices perhaps foreign to you and open you up to the sensation of being in a physically vulnerable state.

2. While topless, have your lover tie your hands and feet together and blindfold you. Then have him give you a massage, as you tell him which body parts to concentrate on. This will open up the titillating world of the unknown. It also will give you a feel for how relaxing life can be in the absence of a "controlling interest" on your part, even as you realize who's *actually* pulling the strings (you). That's the essence of DSRP: yin-yang partnership balance.

3. Recall an occasion in which you found yourself in an argument with someone and were able to quell your aggression and allow the other person to have the last word. How did it make you feel? Recall, too, how the other person reacted to the surprise of your disarming maturity and grace, in ceding the illusion of control to another. Next time you heatedly argue with someone—a friend, a co-worker, a lover, a family member, a sales clerk, a Twitter buddy—and are convinced that you are correct, try a passive approach and surrender. You don't have to capitulate to the argument, just calmly *let it go*, giving the other guy the power s/he needs. Be the submissive and, in the instance, the stronger person.

BUILDING

Erotic Tension

chapter five

I'm a slave for you (here we go now).
I cannot hold it,
I cannot control it.
I'm a slave (it just feels right) for you (it just feels good).
I won't deny it (yeah yeah).
I'm not trying to hide it (baby).
I really want to do what you want me to (uh uh uh).
—BRITNEY SPEARS, "I'M A SLAVE 4 U"

Britney Spears whipped up one psychic orgy of pheromone tension performing her hit single "I'm a Slave 4 U" at the 2001 MTV Video Music Awards.[1] It wasn't so much the words as what she did with them. When she wasn't gyrating and doing other amazing things with her pelvis, she was writhing on the floor or flaunting a live boa draped over her shoulders (giving that albino Burmese python the ride of his/her life, I suspect s/he could tell you). The wantonly sexy performance left the evening's host, Jamie Foxx, visibly (and admittedly) dazed by the palpable heat of her salacious moves, belly-danced in slaaaaaaave-for-you harem girl finery. Rubbing his forehead, Foxx ad-libbed, "I think I have jungle fever," then glanced over at Justin Timberlake (Brit's BF at the time) and muttered, "Lucky man." For this viewer, and likely for the rest of the female viewing audience who "knew her when," the dazing thought was, "Damn! That little ex-Mouseketeer sure has grown up!" (N.b., she was nineteen at the time). I'm no pop star fan but that performance was *hot*. Look it up on YouTube. It was the juice!

And the male viewers? (Foxx, after all, was being paid to be entertainingly emotive.) Were they similarly whelmed? I turn to Mr. H for the guys' take on Britney's vampy profession of slavish devotion.

"It's every man's fantasy to have a beautiful, universally desired woman as his 'slave,'" Mr. H tells me. "The idea that a woman is so turned on by you physically that she will do anything for you is a special thing. It encourages the ego and makes a man feel powerful and strong, and power is the ultimate aphrodisiac. Having a woman try to seduce you and make you her own is attractive because it makes *you* the star in her eyes and boosts your pride/ego/self image. Then, to be anointed—chosen, adored, and served by that woman—it makes a man weak in the knees."

Erotic tension building is a potent tool, as I intend to demonstrate in this chapter. Whether your sexual relationship has gone stale, your guy has a small dinky that you just can't get juiced up about no matter how many times you squeeze your eyes shut and imagine otherwise, or you simply wish to heighten the thrill of your DSRP, there are ways to do a mind-fuck on yourself, to build up your partner to Herculean epic proportions (ahem), and to supersede reality.

Haven't we all, at least once in our lives, perhaps in our long-ago past, felt like that girl in Britney's song, damn near fetishizing some boy-crush? We did it in private, moaning and groaning, overcome by slithery sexual thoughts. And we did it in his presence, powerless to control the mental telegraphing of the glaring, lovesick message: "I'm a *slave* for you." In our adolescent innocence, unpracticed in the ways of the world of courtship, didn't we *so* hope he wouldn't notice (oh, dear), or that, if he did, he wouldn't toy with our emotions, at least not *cruelly*?

Of course! All of the above. We were so young. Now, as healthy and mature adults, choosing that Salome role for dominant and submissive role play is another story altogether. We do so not obsessively, helplessly, but willfully—as Salome played it—in the pursuit of sensual or erotic diversion, in command of our feelings and faculties. I must admit, however, that in revisiting the sexy Brit blowout, I was amused to see all the hot-and-botheredness going on among the studio audience, men *and* women, and was revved up myself. Britney's torrid portrayal of the worshipful slave prompted me to reminisce—from the sanctuary of adulthood—about the first (and last) time I was so hot-obsessed with a boy that I happily/miserably existed in a slave-for-him state, living on passion and desire and not much else. *This* is erotic tension. *This* is DSRP. We can learn from the engulfing dalliances of youth.

The Boy Who ~~Ruined~~ Freed Me (I Never Fell for That Game Again!)

How best to put it? I loved and lost, before I loved and won? Yes, I think that does it. My extended teenage crush was a *bad* boy. In fact, in those days, I was interested *only* in bad boys; I *insisted* on it. No lovesick nice guys from the peer group need apply. Later, older by a few years and a whole bunch wiser—after the Fall, that is—I reappraised the Good Guy (as Lena Dunham, creator of *Girls*, put it, "the guy who doesn't treat [your] heart like monkey meat." *Stinger!*) and began treating myself to men from the Right-Stuff side of the tracks. Wondrously, however, that first *9½ Weeks*-y affair/ordeal offered lessons I have since been able to put to very good use. What we can extract from lessons learned from our bad boy is his formidable bag of tricks, incorporating his persuasive campaign tactics and maneuvers into our play. We gave him a *lot*, no? (Yes!) So now it's time to take? (Yes!) You mad mademoiselles in?

Blushingly, I'll toss you the brief account of my bad boy and his womanizing exploits, for the larger, grander purpose of illustrating some proven ways to bring out the commanding bad boy in your lover.

Seventeen years old. I'd shopped my mother's closet for the right French blazer and the Chinatown sidewalk stalls for a credible fake ID. Thus fitted out and credentialed, I practiced my high-heel walk into a ritzy Madison Avenue lounge patronized by gorgeous name-brand models and sexy rough-stubble-faced bounders—monied riffraff New Yorkers call Eurotrash but whom underage prep school girls fancy for their continental airs. F was a rare find in that milieu. Yes, he had the de rigueur stubble, though he wore it offhandedly, more cocksure Jim Morrison than aristo arriviste. He had attracted an adoring Venus corps of leggy mannequins—*Perfection, thy name is Cover Girl*—all giggling way too rapturously at his every utterance, droll one-liners from the playboy blarney book.

Blast! How could an awkward teen with chin zits, like the weirdo kid from a coming-of-age art film, compete? Somehow, even at the wobbly stage, however, I knew enough to adopt the haughty, dismissive/apathetic act, to ice him. Returning to the bar after a mirror-check in the powder room, head down, acting annoyed, I delivered an imperious "Excuse me, please," as I passed the resplendent clot of the Chosen Few. Whence I pulled out that blue-ribbon, battle-of-the-sexes chess move, lord knows, but impressive, because it worked! I looked up to see a widening of the big blue eyes, a flip of the shiny, straight, thick, black/red rock-god hair, and a twirling around to pay *proper* attention. He was perfect. Perfect. He was Narcissus perfect. The chiseled features of an Irish-American god, with A-list movie star looks and charisma, kicking the likes of Brad Pitt into the ugly brother bin. Charming, hilarious (his brother is a well-known comedian), he had the easy ebb and flow of wiles embedded in his DNA. He was born to make women melt, his greatest talent. F aimed a puff of magic dust straight into my face. Couldn't resist a girl who—huh? what?—actually had the effrontery to ignore him. He was simultaneously stumped and smitten. Casually shooing away the crew of idolizing models, he spent the rest of the night trying to win me over. I stayed chilly—in fact, too scared to pay him attention. For me, the night ended on a high, with Cinderella whisked off in her yellow, metered coach—alone. That clean getaway, I suppose, counts as one face-saving crumb, but if my fairy godmother had really had my back, that matchbook with my scribbled phone number would have spontaneously combusted in F's pants pocket.

He called, of course *(he called!!!!)*, and days later our hot affair took off. Whereas I'd had my puny little moment of triumph that opening night in the lounge, unhappily ever after the victories were all his. I'm telling you, that man shattered my poor little teenage heart into a billion tiny specks of Valentine-red blood splattering over the wretched world of a high school senior. Melodrama, thy name is High School Senior (playing way out of her league). I would wake up and go to sleep praying for a call. When he did call, suggesting a hookup, I'd grab the subway down to his place, on an out-of-my-mind "high" a junkie couldn't buy. The guy "was in my plasma," as Sinatra is said to have wailed after the split with Ava.

How did he do it, turning Chilly Girl into Slave for Him? For starters, it was *his* playground, and he was PlayMaster. I was the kid on both ends of the seesaw and he sat the axis, teetering me up and tottering me down, at will. He was ten years my senior—a fathomless gap at that stage of life—which is to say that, at seventeen and twenty-seven, neither the schoolgirl nor the playboy was mature enough for a serious relationship. While I was a sophisticated child of Manhattan and a rather savvy teenager, I was no match for a seasoned Casanova. Clearly, I never had his "real" number. He had two phone lines—one for *chicks.*

Under his bed and elsewhere around his unkempt Lower East Side apartment, I'd find bras and other undergarments that weren't mine and hadn't been there on my last visit. He would call me, pulling shit like, "You know that diner we went to last week? It burned down two nights ago." "Oh, yeah?" "Yeah. I had this big crush on one of the waitresses, now how the hell am I going to find her?" Half chuckling in mock horror, "What am I going to *do*, Alexis?" Umm, stomach in knots. Stay cool. Hang up. Cry and cry and cry.

He was known as the reigning playboy of the downtown art scene. It was ridiculous. We'd be strolling the LES and chicks—gorgeous, sexy, hip chicks—would run through traffic to wave him down. "F! F!" they'd exult, clutching him passionately and possessively. "Call me, *soon!*" I would stand aside, feigning nonchalance under a shop canopy, while I, like, *died.* On those infrequent days when I was "allowed" to see him, he was charming, tender, affectionate, even nice, and I'd react to the lovemaking like a sex-starved war bride. During our romps in bed, he was coldly dominant, periodically interrupting activities to reiterate, "You know you're too young for me." I would try my best to seduce, play the withholding game myself—"Okay, but I'll only f*** you for a minute," but he refused to be baited. Occasionally, as we sat watching TV, he'd spontaneously take my hand and lead me to his disheveled bed, teasing and withholding till I was ready to *scre-e-e-am.* I still can recall those blitzes of Zeus bolts pumping-pumping-pumping . . . stronger-stronger-stronger through every neuron in my young body each time he spoke, touched me, called me, said my name, bedded me—the rushes so strong that I've been able to recall and relive the thrills of those sensational sessions ever since, employing the firepower in DSRP, erotic tension building, and sensually self-indulgent exercises.

Turnabout Is *Smart* Play

So, yes, F was a hot mess slash rat bastard, but I took from him some first-rate playboy tricks I've found easily adaptable and wildly successful in the sparking up of passions in my normalized, okay-over-it! sexual relationships. F served his purpose. In hindsight, I came to suspect that my extreme infatuation was fired up less by a lust to make him mine than by the aching passion to *become* him: carefree and confident, popular and magnetic, a stardust creature. And once I outgrew (some of) my teenage insecurities and (some of) my teenage egocentricity, once I fit happily into my own skin, that is, I found myself able to apply certain of F's cultivated talents to Alexis-pleasing pursuits. Recalling the triggering mechanisms, I can adopt them to mesmerize my lover, not for cruel purposes but to mutually desired and satisfying ends.

If you are (or ever have been) obsessed with a guy, ask yourself what he has that (1) attracted and continues to hold you, and (2) you feel you lack. Whatever the qualities (maybe simply his MO?), work to develop them in yourself. Whatever the attributes, adopt or even *buy* them. (Long to be prettier? Buy a new nose or chin, as the starlets do.) But did you get the memo? Intelligence is sexy, too. F stuck by my young and foolish self, I'm convinced, because I flaunted not my cutes but my smarts. In fact, F frequently asked my opinion on a book or a piece of artwork, and shortly thereafter I'd hear him publicly expound my opinions as his own. Having grown up in the burbs north of the city, he'd also ask me, the native daughter, to clarify certain social and cultural nuances, poaching my New York state of mind. So, it seemed, at least in part he wanted to be me as well. Too bad I didn't figure that out way back when. All those allowance dollars *wasted!* on designer-brand mascara, unattractively bleeding down the cheeks.

Moving on . . .

How to Turn the Average Joe into the Playmate of Your Fantasies

As prelude to play, you might try reigniting the excitement and a giddy, girly lust for your lover by stirring up some potent psychological friction. Do a con job on yourself, in other words. For maximum hotmeter results for your DSRP, float the illusion that your lover is remote, untouchable—unnervingly, even maddeningly so. All. The. Time.

Again, think back to your teenage crush: the butterflies when you would see him, the explosive thrill when he'd call or give you a passing "hi," the nights you would battle it out between doing your math homework and fantasizing about *him*. The endless conversations you would have with your girlfriends about everything he said and did/didn't do and *does it mean he likes me?!* Oh, swoon, the Juliet days when you were.

in love with being in love. You idolized him, obsessed over him, would have given up a limb just to have him return your affections. That intensity of desire, the sexy stardust, is what you want to bring back into the bedroom. And your partner's illusionary standoffishness, your hungering across the relational divide, is what will fuel the loins and make you surge with thrills when he *deigns* to touch or speak to you during play.

We're going to bring back that pulsing, exhilarating (long-lost?) feeling of lust for your partner, lover, husband. Heighten it to the max. Without getting hurt. We will use the tantalizing lure of forbidden fruit to stoke your fire and then fan those flames to set him ablaze. Sound like fun? Grab a pencil and let's go.

Note: This is better and more assuredly and handily played out in the familiar territory of a secure, committed relationship, in which you know and trust your costar and can put your faith in his amorous impulses. But if you feel you can trust your gut with a newer crush, you'll find that the passion-priming routines pay dividends, as well. (We don't want any monkey-meat hearts or mascara'd cheeks.)

Like other trusty pointers from the DSRP playbook, these plotlines are most successfully executed according to script. There's always room for improv (you'll see that inspiration starts to come naturally, as you move through the scenes), but *do* keep your focus on the hoped-for sensational climax. (Grinny face.) Proceed carefully. Pick the strategies you like, and try to consider even the ones you feel might be embarrassing. Ignore the ones you feel might hurt you emotionally in any way! Posh girls don't play that game. So off you go!

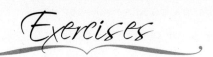
Exercises

1. Limit contact.

2. Playing to your insecurities and his strengths and attractive qualities, have him tell you a story, in detail, of an instance in which a girl desperately wanted him and he did not, or could not, return her affections. Bolster your illusion of your play partner as a bad boy.

3. Instruct him to respond to your communications—calls, texts, emails, beeps, Facebook posts, tweets, smoke signals, and all else—75 percent less than is his usual pattern.

4. Carry around one of your lover's sweaty T-shirts or store it in your lingerie drawer. Smell it every day, as frequently as possible. What? Why? Better you listen to a social scientist than to me: "Maybe it's not similar interests, horoscope signs, looks, or proximity that make women and men fall in love. . . . Subtle chemical signals, or pheromones, have long been known to draw pairs together within the same species. . . . In the first 'sweaty T-shirt' experiment, a Swiss zoologist, Claus Wedekind, set up a test of women's sensitivity to male odors."[2]

    Pheromone, BTW, sounds like *saxophone*. Think sexy music jazzing up the sex drive. *C'est oooolala!*

5. Have him point out girls he finds hot—in public, on TV, and on the Internet—or ask him which girls he finds sexy, and why. Maybe your best friend? Well, that could build some hot competitive tension, though you may want to refrain from suggesting he act on his attraction in that particular case (!). Swinging has ruined many relationships, in which partners naïvely overestimated their open-mindedness and tolerance. It can be icing on the DSRP cake, but I'd reserve that risky venture for a time way into the game, when advanced-play couples know the ropes and their psychological limits.

6. Risky one—be warned! Have him strike up a flirty Facebook conversation with a girl he finds hot; ideally, she lives far away, i.e., across the continent or ocean. Playing fair, he should state he's in a relationship but (to throw out just one idea) wants to chat in the interest of a mutual friend. Have him let you read the emails and forward all flirtations to you. All the she-said/he-said. This is sure to create some playful jealously—though is perhaps a safe pursuit for no longer than a month or so (or not at all, if you feel one ping of a bad gut feeling about it).

7. Give him BJs in clean public and party-house bathrooms or, for the more reserved Posh Girl, in the bathroom of your/his apartment or house. Then have him leave. Take fifteen minutes before reuniting.

8. Sleep in separate rooms. Put him on the couch. Or, if you live separately, retire for the night to your own digs—for a week. Better yet, a month!

9. Have him bring you close to orgasm and call a halt, on ten separate sexual romp occasions. Politely end the romp and leave the room. Separate immediately afterward. Then masturbate alone following his departure. In shared living quarters, go sleep on the couch.

10. Have your partner/dominant withhold a certain kind of favored sexual action, and then relent and perform it. All the tensions and anxiety buildup associated with unfulfilled desire will be suddenly relieved. What would you bet that neurologists could tell us that oxytocin—or whatever that happy sauce hormone is called—comes flooding out at that precise moment?

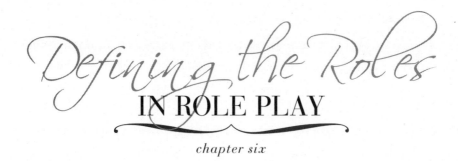

Defining the Roles
IN ROLE PLAY

chapter six

Sugar, I want to know you, know you inside out.
Mystery surrounds you, got to figure it out.
Driving downtown to your house, your lights are never on.
You got me hooked, I wanna drown.
Without your hand I'm going down.
Who's your man? Who's your man? Who's your man?
—INXS, "REMEMBER WHO'S YOUR MAN"

So, *Sugar*, let's help the guy out, turn on some *lights* already! He's *begging* for answers, poor little monkey. You foxes just know he's not as savvy as you, and still you expect him to read that mystery mind of yours?

You're the one who read *that book*, no? Got the frisky notions, decided to put them into play? That would make it your production, yours to stage and to *sell*. First on your to-do list, then: Decide and define who it is that you want your role-play dominant to "be." Once you have a definable character to dangle before him, you can boldly declare your intentions and shrewdly and methodically start the molding process that will bring him to life as your dom.

Ask yourself some questions to help you pin down the identity of the characters in your role-playing scene. For example, who's the man you want pulling your strings? A deadly cold, utterly detached dominant, with you as the object pet, existing solely for his pleasure? The "daddy dom" (as the good doctor said, all girls crave a father's attention), doting on you, disciplining you, babying you? The master with a devoted you as his slave object (called objectification, described in chapter 4)? The criminal/intruder dom aggressive, an unforgiving invader savoring his captive's alarm and discomfort? The well-bred gentleman whose commanding presence is quite enough to ensure he gets his way? (Does the name Christian come to mind?) Or, for a more personally invasive proposition guaranteed to heighten the intensity factor: Cue the blackmailer dom, the extortionist who knows just where your buttons are and delights in pushing them; humiliating and mentally torturing you, mercilessly, slowly, deliciously; pushing you to the edge of your emotional breaking point, where you'll do *anything* to stop the pain and suffering.

Just as you know when you've found the *perfect* little black dress, you'll know when you've come up with the perfect role-play persona for your man. It's waaay easier to get into character, block out your responsive role play, and set up your scene (covered in the next chapter) if you nail down the characters first. Most important is that you flesh out the personality of the dominant player, as it is he who will fulfill your fantasies.

If you're having trouble conceiving an identity for your costar, go back and read your erotic story. Is there a dominant character profile mentioned above that fits the description of the fantasy dom in your story? If not, work your imagination to invent your own dominant persona. It may help to Google through your own fiction memory bank to recall a compelling character from a story, a novel, or a film and tailor your DSRP partner to that memorable guy.

As you refine the character of your dominant partner, continue to ask yourself questions:

1. How does your fantasy dom speak to you and handle you sexually? Meanly? Aggressively? Menacingly? Dismissively? Firmly? Softly but domineeringly?

2. How does he "punish" you? Harshly? Reluctantly? Physically or emotionally?

3. Does he show any mercy? (If the answer is no, he still must respect your hard limits, of course.)

4. Do you wish to feel afraid of him? Or would you rather see him as an authority figure, firm and controlling but not frightening?

The Spill

The easiest, and in the long run the best, way to get what you want is to be upfront in portraying the character you'd like him to role-play. Describe the figure you have chosen—you might even give him a name—and engage your partner in the process with questions only he can answer, e.g., what appeals, what he can handle. Describe the character's personality and give your partner loose examples of how your fantasy dominant might react in defined role-play actions.

For example, in speaking to your lover, you might say: "The guy I fantasize about is modeled on [name of character] in [title of book or movie]." (If it's a novel he hasn't read or a film he hasn't seen, give a brief synopsis and a character description.) "He speaks gently but firmly and undresses me slowly, coldly teasing me as I'm being disrobed. He punishes me only when I refuse to perform a sexual act he requests or when I struggle while being tied up or 'ravished.' He punishes me, not harshly but firmly, through such acts as pulling my hair, spanking me, or pinching my nipples, until I give in. Or he brings me close to orgasm and then stops."

Or you might say: "He's very aggressive and scary. He doesn't hurt me, but I see him as a cold-blooded intruder and sense that he is capable of hurting me. He manhandles me, talks dirty, and says insulting things, calling me a whore, bitch, slut, because he can tell I've 'sucked a lot of c***.' He warns that if I don't do what he says, he will slap my 'c***-teaser face.' He follows through on the threat when I 'act out' or refuse to follow his orders."

This is the kind of information I give my partner, but you may wish to go further. You can read him parts of your story or passages from the book you've cited, or have him watch the movie you have in mind. Then you can say, "Now *this* is what I want!" Go into detail if he asks. *Never* ignore a question he poses, however embarrassing, because in skirting the issues, you risk two things: not getting exactly what you want from him and, worse, leaving critical judgment calls to him. The devil is in the details—*know that!*

Pose questions that will prompt him to do a little soul-searching on his own. For example: "Assuming the role of [character name or type], will you be able to address me roughly and behave in an aggressive manner? Not really aggressively, then, but firmly? If the scene requires that you deliver verbal taunts and humiliating put-downs, could you handle that? How about tying me up? Roughing me up a bit?"

I've Looked at Life from Both Sides Now . . . Gathering Useful Intelligence from the Dominant's POV

During my brief and enlightening (is that the word? yes, *enlightening* will do) stint as a dominatrix, my clients—roughly a quarter were submissive women and the rest were men—succeeded in shaping me into their ideal archetypal domme through suggestion: verbal hints and, during play, subtle uses of body language. They were practiced insiders and they expected me to "get it." Usually I did. Although my sessions (that's the pro-domme term for "role play hours") were nonsexual, the demands of my subs were the same as if we'd been lovers: All wanted me to behave as a distinct dominant character. A common approach for subs requesting a session was to address me via email with explicit descriptions of the types of scenes they wanted. They communicated what they wished me to say and do, often through detailed scripts. From all that, I was able to discern not only their persona but my own, as well: Mommy Domme, Mommy Dearest Domme, Haughty Uptown Girl, Mean Girl, Demanding Glamour Girl, Female Bitch Boss, Prison Warden—the list is as boundless as your ingenuity.

In other words, effective communication patterns are equally important to subs and dommes/doms, in the conveying and comprehending of wishes. Reading the clues and getting the message, however, doubtlessly is easier for women than it is for men—that female intuition thing is no figment—so patience and perseverance are rewarded here. You do want to be sure he's "hearing" the news you're conveying. If he's receptive to the proposal, he'll feel an equal investment in the preplanning dialogue. After all, he's your partner and he wants to please you, right? (Not right? So what do we do with a spiffy pair of heels that looks hot but doesn't quite fit? Uh-huh.) Most likely, the hunter instinct will kick in, and he'll work for that ego boost promised through the act of sexually satisfying you. Thus, he will make the mental effort to track and follow your footprints along the trail toward your tempting new playground.

Here's an idea that should drive home the significance of the shifting sands of dominant/submissive dynamics.

Now you see it: The dom is calling the shots, bending the sub to his will, exercising his male prerogative—in short, he's the taker.

Now you don't: Who started this role-play business? Who laid down the terms? Who's calling the shots? In short, she's wearing the pants.

If you're a cat person, you'll recognize the dynamic right off: A cat enters the house and straightaway begins to train us to give her exactly what she wants and needs. Willingly, eagerly, we answer; we feed her, house her, call ourselves her "owner," and introduce her as "my pet." But is there a cat keeper in the world who doesn't acknowledge to Kittycat herself, "You master, me slave"? And there you have it.

So, down with the misapprehension that female sexual submissives are not in the driver's seat, not in control. As the sub, you create and mold him (*your* dominant!) to your specifications. To serve your fantasy, not his. To be your puppet of pleasure. And now that we've settled that, we won't talk of it again.

Herewith, Some Additional Tricks of the Trade

Give hints to get the play action back on *your* course, when things go awry.

When I was a pro domme, what seemed to work really well for me, without spoiling the scene, was learning to read the subs' clues along the way as to what they wanted from me. They were experienced masters of the verbal and nonverbal clue, and I learned a lot from them. If, for instance, I was being too aggressive, the sub, his/her face tensing up, might say, "You are very strict" (hint, hint). That was my clue to chill. If I was not being aggressive enough, the sub might say, "I know what I did was bad . . . what are you going to do to me? Please don't _____ me." The words, almost seductive in tone, along with the telling body language—a happy face, an alert, buoyant, eager posture—were a very clear cue to ramp up the action, as the sub was effectively hinting.

In my own play, I rarely have to give hints, as I'm a goody-good girl and am always *veddy veddy* explicit in detailing the character type I want him to be, what I like and do not like, and what I might do if coaxed (stretching my soft limits).

Now, hard and soft limits can change every day or over time, just as your fantasy dominant persona may slip between characters. You may be in the mood for one character and scene tonight and crave something more, or less, intense the day after tomorrow. He shouldn't be expected to read your mind. Communicate your fresh desires and be prepared to give him some non-scene-breaking pointers as play progresses.

There's a role-play exercise common in acting class, based on the idea of conflict: One person wants something from his or her scene partner, who wants another thing altogether. At first, student actors tend to go full-on aggressive, a tactic guaranteed to end at stalemate—no one gives in. Eventually, one of the actors (in my experience, it's always the female) figures she'll get more with honey than with tough talk and wisely plays to the endgame. She may, for example, express her desire for the said object or result and then shrug it off, nonchalantly indicating that there will be no angry words if she doesn't get her way. Now, the male actor knows his job here is not to give in, but what happens most times is interesting: He begins to *want* to give it to her and is even kind to her and empathetic to her restrained frustration. I see that acting scene outcome as a win for the submissive (and so does the teacher). The objective is irrelevant. The trick is to make the other person feel like a schmuck for being so stubborn, dismissive, and unreasonable. It's not necessary to play games; better to be sincere and kind, and most men will buckle.

You don't want to get pissy or irritated if he's iffy about playing your fantasy dominant character or if he doesn't score on his first time out of the chute at the role-play rodeo. Remember, it's about the endgame. Be expressive and gentle. Calm and kind. Honey not vinegar, dahlings. Much more posh.

Common Myths

While honing your ideas for your fantasy dominant character, it's best to keep your partner's personality in mind. There are several common myths about how various male personality types will perform in bed, and most of them are false.

My lover is a tough guy.
He'll have no problem fitting into the aggressive dominant role.
THINK AGAIN.

My lover is sensitive and not so manly . . . and he's a bit submissive in life.
He'll have a very hard time being my perfect dominant.
THINK AGAIN.

I've found that the sensitive artist and metrosexual types of men I've dated *love, love, love* an opportunity to turn the tables, play the dominant, and dominate me. The rough-and-toughie badass dudes were scared to be "mean" to me in bed, scared they'd "hurt" me.

Role play often reflects the principle of the yin and yang. The submissive in bed is usually (not always) dominating in life. The guy who kicks ass as a dominant in bed is usually (not always) a bit submissive in "matters of the heart." A man may be cock of the walk in his peer group, may exercise the power of his position, his riches, or his muscles, but I'm always amused to find that, deep down, the swashbuckler's really not tough, but a bit of a softy.

Interesting, no?

What I'm saying is, don't assume that your lover will play true to form, based on your perceptions of his persona, the personality he fronts to the world. He will play his part—the part you've conceptualized— with flying f'ing colors, or he'll flop, with flying f'ing colors. Be prepared for surprise.

A COMMON DILEMMA: *WHAT IF MY man is rough and tough in the world but refuses to be tough with me in bed?*

I've come up against this problem on occasion, myself. By way of example: I had a longtime fling with an American reporter whose crime beat included coverage of Al-Qaeda and the New York scene, street criminals and mobsters. Physically, he was incredibly brave, having interviewed America's nemesis terrorist with goons aiming machine guns at his face. He (legally) carried a gun. He was a big, bawdy, manly man who drank manly drinks at Elaine's (the NYC bar/salon patronized by tough guys and writers and tough-guy writers, which I mentioned in chapter 2). A girl might reasonably have assumed the guy would be firm, controlling, and overpowering in bed, but . . . nope, nope, nope. He was a sensitive li'l pussycat in bed, def not what I'd signed up for, darn it! One night I noticed his gun on his bedside table, picked it up, jokingly pretended to be a femme fatale, pointed it at him, and said . . . can't recall, probably something really stupid, trying to play the part. I don't know how he did it, but he "handled the situation," stayed chill. I put it down and he "ravaged" me (meaning, it was like he hadn't seen a girl in twenty years). I recall turning around and . . . the gun was just gone. Poof! I'd given him a little role-play push along the lines of "I'm being extremely bad. *Now* will you please dominate me in bed, play-rape me?" Jeez. Where's the toughie guy?

Now, I'm not recommending that you play with guns, kiddies. *Noooooooo!* That was me being totally idiotic and irresponsible. But there are other ways to find a serviceable way to get through to him . . . playfully.

Using body language, continued. Now, the lead player in the former tale lived on the Upper East Side of Manhattan. Downtown, on East Third Street, I was having a concurrent fling with a man I'll call X, a bigwig member of the Hells Angels. A serious badass, he was big, hulking, terrifying, with long, straight, blond hair and deadly cold blue eyes that wouldn't let anyone in. A Viking Genghis Khan. But. He was a graduate of a prestigious art school, a photographer celebrated for his documenting of the biker world. He was not a chauvinist. In fact, when I'd snap at him (I'm snappy), he would say, "You think I have no feelings."

Anyway, you wouldn't be off the mark to assume, "Oh, this time she's got a guy who will dominate the holy hell out of her in bed." Nope. *Sighs*. He was *more* the gentle pussycat than that lionhearted reporter. Shoot!

Until, that is, I coaxed the beast out of him in bed. And how did Missy Frost do *that*? It was odd, as if each of us recognized the type-A alpha hunter creature in the other. As if he sensed that an invade-and-conquer would break my pride and break the spell. As if he had this bratty, high-spirited thoroughbred and liked seeing her running free around his biker clubhouse.

One fated night in his hunter lair, we argue. It becomes a battle of takedowns between two stubborn-ass tempers. Who knows how things started, but I snap. I snap on a "Filthy Few" badge member (the "Filthy Few" being a badge to tip off other bikers that this man is a skilled brawler). My temper flares to a height rarely seen. The unfortunate few who have witnessed this state have described my eyes looking like "a wildcat gone ballistic"—as in, I'm not there anymore. Those wild feline eyes don't pierce but blaze, and I cat-swipe a curse across his face: "You're fucked. You are going down for something *soon!* Know that!" With X, the parry and thrust is delivered through the ice-blue eyes, not wild but warrior cold. His angry beast is surface-calm, ready to spring but betraying nothing. Sitting, waiting, with a frozen-wall stare that chills your core, mocks a hellcat's fire. Cats hate cages and, as I'm feeling trapped, my claws strike against his hulking warrior frame. My involuntary feline instinct is to break the icy death stare with the ice pick of my hand, jolting him from the locked-in terror hold he has on me. I strike. We both pause. Not a flicker of rage escapes the frozen void. I am fucked.

I know I can't turn things around or try to leave because when you back down before a beast of prey, you ask for death. I'm panicking silently so as not to show the weakness that would invite the kill. We stare. This carnivorous slayer is NOT. GOING. TO. MOVE. He's waiting for me to acknowledge fear and to submit. What the hell is he going to do? I cannot let him win. I'm too scared I've just awakened the X. I don't know, dark ice sociopath, as biker legend would have it. My feline body goes into hunter stance lockdown, my eyes fixed on his, my nails lightly tapping the (shudder) coffin he uses for a coffee table. With every claw tap I'm wildly exhuming subconscious survival instincts. I can't be nice now, it's gone too far; he'll sense weakness and attack. I start to cackle, laughing sardonically as a way to break the ice, then lose the Cheshire cat smile, and in a fluid yet powerful jaguar motion, thrust my head back to expose my neck. I shift my eyes down seductively and let my bottom lip drop as I exhale with a low purring roar and gracefully shift my shoulder forward. I reach out my hand and run my feline fingers down his chest, letting my half-mast cat eyes drift away from his kill stare, going for coy, not sensual. My actions, I can tell, have him off-balance, like he's staring at a female cat. She comes over, he pets her, then she scratches him. She rubs her head on him and begins to twitch her tail. Is she going to strike again or purr? My instincts are telling me that mystery will throw him off. Few females can tap into their feline prowess, but I am a feline-humanoid. Reared with (and by) cats, no siblings.

X pulls an assassin move, grabs the back of my wrist, flips my arm around, and twists it behind my back, forcing my body against his so that I'm again staring into the void of his eyes. Ahhhh, another manipulative, deep, and sultry kitty breath. I'm terrified. Is he going to kill me or f*** me? Honestly, given his rage, I'm not sure. A split second is all he'd need to execute a one-two pounce and pulse stroke. Figure it's not likely I'm worth a kill. But maybe he has snapped, too?

My claw-tap tail-switch thinking has been quelled. All is still. A stare lock. I feel if I kiss him, he'll see that as obvious manipulation and not trustworthy, female capitulation through wiles. So, as he continues to pin my arm behind me, I fling my blond mane to the side and strike! Bite his ear, but carefully. He grabs my hair, pulling my teeth from his flesh, and I instinctively push my body closer to his and with my other hand grab his long blond lion locks. This jars him and he pushes me onto the couch, pouncing on top of me. I pull my free arm over my head as if to signal kill, take, chew away. But I know that in this position he could opt for the real kill. The man vs. woman kill. Still staring through me with icy sociopath eyes, he clutches my breast. I arch my back like a cat being stroked. He pulls down my shiny black yoga pants and I undo his heavy black leather belt and cold metal zipper. He is mine. I am his. We go at it like untamed feline and cruel assassin. Every thrust-thrust-thrust gets less aggressive and forceful, as I'm taking each beat of his manhood into my gripping void, clenching him tighter and tighter so as not to let him go, just as his killer stare locked in my attention. Something about his kill-or-fuck eyes scares me into a frenzy and I go cat-crazy insane. I'm jolting, screaming, kicking, and clawing, seizing the opportunity to go batshit wild and release every terror-stifled, pent-up animal impulse to explode. Nobody wins and nobody conquers. What happens is what happens when two carnivores hit it.

X's blond hair is matted with mine. His eyes are now relaxed and meat-drunk, like he's fed on my blood and is done. I slip out and walk half naked in a confident stride to the bathroom. I weep-cry, careful not to let him hear. It's the nature of the cat beast that wild rage turns to wild outpouring of emotion. My nerves need calming, so I cry. Then I splash the green cat eyes, fling open the bathroom door, and demand, "I'm hungry, I want a roast beef sandwich." X looks up like a satisfied lion tamer and hustles to get an all-night diner menu. I slink to the scene-of-the-crime couch and nestle in, tilting my head back on the arm rest, neck exposed, waiting for my roast beef.

That was many moons ago. I knew nothing of DSRP or, as they say, BDSM in full. But I felt my way through what I saw as primal body language. If words fail or his understanding of your words fails, turn to body language. It's smooth, clean, and very hard to misinterpret. If you are not naturally physically expressive and have a hard time translating your thoughts through gestures and movements, then try a dance class or a yoga class. Visit the zoo and watch how animals stretch and move to interact. Their communication through movement is honest, pure, and never misleading. We are told to embrace certain social conditioning rules through "proper" movements. Remember, you are a sexual creature. We are all. Physical action results in returned physical action. In DSRP, this equation works in shaping your man into your fantasy character.

Exercises

1. Revisit the erotic story you wrote for the second exercise in chapter 1. Pay attention to how you described your fantasy male dominant and his actions. Or envision a DRSP scene from a movie or book that excited you and, if you're plucking from fiction, then fixate on the male dominant in the scene and ask yourself what attracts you to him and his persona.

2. Now write down, or simply envision, three adjectives that capture the actions of your fantasy male dominant (e.g., aggressive, shocking, forceful, controlling, sensual, steady, determined), and tailor your developing dom profile to those qualities that elicited favorable responses in you.

3. Now this one takes a little time and is not easy, but it's worth the effort. Why? Because it will help you get inside your head, almost like hacking into your own subconscious.

   SO DIG: Write twenty sentences for me, as follows. Drawing from concrete and abstract thoughts on your new working model, describe your ideal sexual dominant. Imagine you are writing him as a character, conceiving him, and try to portray him in full. You'll see, things get really interesting at about the ten mark. I felt as if I started digging deep at eleven. It seems that once you commit to the written word, it's almost as if you cast a spell, embedding a vignette of your ideal into your head. And as you begin to project those thoughts, the profile of your character will manifest itself. Sounds like sorcery, I know, but I see the process as less *Witches of Eastwick* than Oprah's "vision board" (you might Google that). (An aside: this exercise is equally applicable to a search for your "ideal mate" and can help you slice through the crop of dating game contenders.)

4. Show the list of your favored DSRP dominant characteristics to your lover and discuss. If you find that too embarrassing, simply use hints about your preferences to begin shaping his role and his moves. My own inclination is to be direct, as it's the fastest way to get what you want from the chap. Most men find sex talk hot, so make sure your "spill" is full of colorful detail and racy possibility.

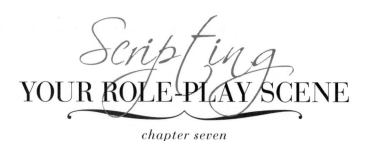

YOUR ROLE-PLAY SCENE

chapter seven

Where any barmaid can be a star maid
If she dances with or without a fan
Hooray for Hollywood
—"HOORAY FOR HOLLYWOOD"
(RICHARD WHITING/JOHNNY MERCER)

How do they *do* it, those Hollywood makers of magic? They take over the back lot of a studio, cobble together a grand forties night-club, put a fitted white tux on the star, a classy blond on his arm, cue the piano, and call it *Casablanca*. Hooray, indeed! We know it's not *really* real, but those scene-making pros make us *believe!* So, how *do* they do it?

One tip, and a valuable thought to hold as you embark on scripting your scene, comes from a book on the making of *Casablanca*, in a discussion of the many artistic accommodations those H'wood producers were obliged to make. "Verisimilitude," the author wrote, "was more important than truth anyway."[1] Good word that, for our purposes: "the appearance or semblance of truth or reality" (according to Collins

English Dictionary) is what's really going to sell us on our own fantasies. We will script our scene and then we'll make do with inspired choices of convincing details to provide the truthiness.

Of course, we don't have the resources or know-how of seasoned filmmakers, and in staging our own productions we may have to cut corners, but making do is part of the fun in exercising creativity. No matter how implausible the storyline (Ilsa walking into Rick Blaine's nightclub, in Morocco, anyone?), a few strategically chosen props and some ambient mood-makers can buy you your reality. You'll see.

One thing before we begin: If you decide to go the loosey-goosey route in scripting your scene, meaning you choose to go with a barebones script that allows for much spontaneous improv, be sure at least to communicate and come to full agreement with your partner regarding your hard and soft limits, physical and verbal, and the type of dominant character you desire, e.g., aggressive or gentle but firm. Also—important!—establish your safe word and/or red-flag body gesture/action.

First off, I will divulge a real-life scene, from my own experience, for which there was medium scripting. After that, I will toss you a mock script for a fully imagined scene. And finally, I will propose other scenarios, along with ideas on how to script them.

Alexis Goes First:
How I Met Mr. H, a Sample Role-Play Scene

I first met Mr. H years ago after stumbling upon his bondage guide blog. I emailed him fishing for a possible role-play encounter but dissembled and portrayed myself as simply wanting more info on his techniques. As a professional dominatrix at the time and coming from an all-girls (extremely uptight) prep school, it was embarrassing even to accept my fantasies of being tied and/or ravaged and dominated by a male. With a little liquid courage, I rallied the nerve to contact him and free myself from some conditioned restraints.

What the hell was I doing?

I wasn't forward enough to straight-out propose a meeting, and maybe more, but through my breezy emails he caught on that likely I was looking to "try" his techniques with him. I received an email from him saying, "Would you like to have coffee and discuss further?" It seemed like a simple and harmless commitment, so I agreed. As I sat waiting for him at a New York City coffee lounge (downtown/upscale), I was terrified that he'd show up and be some perv or creep.

How would I politely brush him off in the flesh?

I don't know if he was intentionally late, hoping to raise my anxiety and thus gain the upper hand, but it worked. The front door swung open again, and this time I felt it was *him*. He was dressed in a black Prada-looking shirt and slick pants but had an arty edge to his gait, sort of a playboy-smooth groove in his step. He was dark-haired and tall and had the physique of an Olympic swimmer. Through his sunglasses, he panned the room and knew instantly I'd be his victim. His consensual victim. Perhaps my nervously shifting eyes gave it away? "Alexis . . ." he said.

"Yes, hi," I answered, and off he went, at first slow and friendly with small talk and then artfully coaxing me along, gradually making me reveal what bondage acts and scenes in his blog had most appealed. There was a natural attraction between us, aside from the common S&M interest. He said, or rather smoothly slipped in, "Might I invite you to try a scene with me?" I tried to be casual and not seem scared and accepted his offer. We picked a date to meet at my apartment.

Blackout.

My apartment. Oh God, oh God, there wasn't enough Bordeaux in the world to calm my nerves, my fears, and the pulsing inner voice that said, "Properly reared girls like you simply do not engage in this kind of behavior." But, thankfully, my curiosity and repressed, now exploding, fantasies won the "good girl/naughty girl" inner battle. Pacing around my apartment, primping and preening, trying to hold a hot blow-dryer as a glass of wine teetered on the side of the sink. *Ding-ding-ding!* My cell went off.

Fuck!

No time, no time to answer. I looked at the display and saw it was *him*. He was sending me a text right before he arrived, asking if I had any formal businesswoman attire. I respond via text, "Yes," then quickly started rummaging through my closet like a fifteen-year-old getting ready for a first rendezvous with a boy.

Dressed in my finest pro biz duds, I let Mr. H into my realm, which quickly became his realm. He came in and immediately, coldly yet not aggressively, asked me to sit in a chair with my eyes closed. I did as asked.

(Pause tape. Okay, here we go to the embarrassing, nitty-gritty, hot details of my first sexual submission to a, well yes, the cliché: tall, dark, and handsome stranger. Right, roll tape . . .)

He lifted my skirt and just left me there. Then he tied my hands behind the chair with pantyhose he'd apparently found in one of my drawers, already revealing his all-knowingness, expert skills, and finesse. I had a hard time submitting. If I didn't put up a teeny bit of a fight, would he think I was a slut? That's what I feared, so I struggled. He said into my ear that if I continued to struggle, he would slap my face. It was up to me. I relented, and he proceeded to blindfold me with another found garment. He took off my pantyhose and tried to gag me by stuffing a pair of panties into my mouth. I freaked out, pleading that I had claustrophobic issues with not being able to breathe through my mouth (communication in action—my early lesson in the importance of presetting limits!), so he said, "Well then, you'll have to let me do something to you." Again, coming events were in my hands. I thought about it and said, "Okay, fine." He placed a hard, square, plastic object between my private parts and panties . . . what the hell was it?

I then heard a ring from a cell phone between my legs, each ring accompanied by a vibration. He kept calling, which was stimulating me, as he could tell from my heavy breathing and moistening-up. He proceeded to stop, start, stop, start, leaving me desperate for more vibration. I was getting aroused and frustrated simultaneously. He began to grope my breasts, and as I was already turned on, I welcomed the manhandling, the pinching of my nipples. I began to speak, and he warned that if I didn't shut up, he'd stick my wet panties into my mouth. He then began to dance his finger around my opening, and it was pure sexual torture. In a good way. The vibrating/fondling and the dancing finger continued for what seemed like an hour. Okay, okay, he got me, jeez. He then told me he was going to sit on my couch and watch TV and that if I wanted him to fuck me, I would have to crawl on my knees to him, rub my head on his leg, and beg. He said, "You have to say, 'I want you to fuck me,' or no satisfaction will be coming your way."

Now this pissed me off! Here I was, Domme Dietrich, expected to crawl to a man and, what's this, begging for sex? Too humiliating and embarrassing for this pro domme! On the other hand, sitting there all ready and frustrated . . . I, uhhhh, got over it. I crawled all right, but with head held high, and as I rubbed my face against his leg I bit it in a burst of professional pride. He said, "Oh, now you're really in trouble. You have a choice: panties in your mouth with tape or sucking my . . ."

Eenie meenie, both repugnant thoughts, but, given the choice and wanting more, I closed my eyes and agreed to deep throat. He was right. It did turn me on further. To my mind, blowjobs are the *ultimate submissive act*. In the past, as I've mentioned, I'd tell BFs to see a hooker if they wanted a BJ, that I wouldn't mind (meant it). That day, with Mr. H, was the first BJ I had ever given. I was a BJ virgin. Miss Prep Cold-Fish Priss no more. I suppose the sexual frustration he so cunningly and wickedly aroused in me overrode my socially conditioned compunctions, and my brain went *off* (i.e., in the right orbit frontal cortex, if you're taking notes). My awakened kinky urges flashed red lights for *on*! But old habits die hard, and in another burst of ego pride, I bit down on his manhood. Well, somebody's Bible got it right: pride goes before a fall and haughtiness before destruction. He immediately, with eerie calm, whipped me about and started to spank me. I squealed and squirmed and his fingers slid down to resume their evil dance, slipping around on the wet dance floor, to hide embarrassment under a metaphor.

Finally, in a frenzy of blood-pounding sexual angst, I relented, went all the damn way: "I want you to fuck me!" [Note: Before this encounter, I was so prim and reserved that, even after working as a pro domme, I couldn't bring myself to speak the words *fuck*, *fingering*, or *cum*, so that "Fuck me!" marked a life-changing breakthrough. If my prep school, plaid-uniformed, straight-haired girlfriends could have seen what a wanton fiend I was being, I would have died in mortification. Without such audience, however, I continued to beg, "I want you to fuck me!"]

He laid me down on the floor and repeated the finger dance with what I felt to be a monster in size—guess that's why he was so confident in his role play! He was huge and impressive! He demanded again, "Tell me you want me to fuck you." I waited, and then in an exasperated gasp blurted it out. He slipped his monster into me and it cured all my repression, right there on the (G-) spot! I asked him to untie my hands as our body weight was pressing on them, and he said, "Okay, but I'm going to have to stick a finger up your backside."

I freaked out. *No, no, no!* But then . . . as the motion of his monster sent me into sexual pleasure overload blackout, I acquiesced. He slipped a finger in, and I tensed up. He politely took it away. That invasion, after a few seconds of processing, made me even hotter. I arched up to kiss him, and he answered arch with arch, in polite tones: "I don't kiss whores." But I recognized it as role play, and the name-calling brought me even closer to climax. When he sensed that I was on the brink of exploding into a huge O, he stopped and told me to beg him to continue, saying that unless I wanted him to stop, I'd have to do something really juicy, risqué. Shocking myself, I did.

In my sexual blackout, I bit it again. He slapped me across the face and said, "If you struggle again, I'll fuck you up the ass." I was such a good girl after that threat, and it didn't take long for me to cum-bust into the most momentous orgasm I'd ever had. OMG! Afterward, he carefully dismounted and left the room.

I lay there, catching my breath and digesting the whole crazy scene. About fifteen minutes later he returned to untie me and offered to get me a glass of water. I asked if he would bring me a cigarette and a light as well. Considering that he'd just "defiled" me, I felt I had the upper hand now. Back in princess mode, I made him dote on me and serve me as he exulted in the guilty pleasure of having "controlled" and "tortured" me.

He became my virtual butler, and I enjoyed feeling like a sexy and pleasured old-school Hollywood star. I don't remember what we talked about, but he spent the night and, like a gentleman, made me feel secure the next morning. I've been seeing Mr. H on and off ever since.

Summing up, I'd say this real-life scenario had it all: surprise, the thrill of the new, and an intuitive dom who correctly sized up what I needed and wanted from an introductory DSRP scene and *gave it to me!* I escaped the hold of my implanted upper-crust-upbringing rules and became *me*, tuning out the clucking noises of my judgmental social circle. I felt freed, and a new confidence tingled inside. The liberation felt damn good.

The Fantasy Robbery

One of the most popular role-play fantasies is the robbery scene. I'll let Mr. H explain the appeal.

Mr. H: Here's a confession I hear repeatedly from female readers—and once, I confess, as a shameless eavesdropper to a rush-hour subway conversation between two young career women discussing DSRP robbery scene entry techniques from my own blog. (They were close readers, I must say!) All have fantasized about the frightening experience of being robbed. Most commonly, musings on the robbery scenario come from women who've earlier expressed curiosity about the concept of bondage and the tantalizing possibility of integrating the practice into the robber/victim scene, to heighten the players' sense of reality.

The account they sketch has them coming home after work to interrupt a robbery-in-progress, or being caught off guard while in the apartment. They've all shuddered through the eleven o'clock news report of the woman down the street whose home was invaded by a thug, who left her bound, gagged, and clearly rattled. With odd fascination, all imagined themselves in the victim's shoes and wondered what they would feel being menaced and forcibly restrained at the hands of a total stranger (no common criminal, I must add, but invariably cast from *You Will Meet a Tall Dark Stranger*). The women who shared their interest in the robbery thing are a diverse club of humans. Thirtysomething bankers, college students, lawyers, church girls, homemakers, teachers, goths, and even a police officer (!!!) all have told me in great detail how they've thought about the great "what if" and how excitedly they found themselves reacting to the prospect. Of course, nobody really wants to risk actual physical harm and the loss of property. What they do want is a shake-up to their daily routine, life interrupted, to live the fantasy of being overpowered, being compelled to surrender and reveling in the sublime pleasure of submission.

THE STAGED BREAK-IN IS ONE OF the easier and more fulfilling "full-force" fantasies one can indulge, as it takes place within the confines of one's own walls. If special care is taken to protect both parties (the submissive physically and the dominant legally), this kind of game can deliver a unique punch (to the senses, that is) for both parties. As old as the bondage ritual itself, the break-in fantasy allows for role play to be bolstered by the attendant feeling of "reality" that does not present in a dungeon setting. Too, the thrill factor way outstrips and outclasses the simple bedroom bondage game in the DSRP stakes. Of course, this type of hunter-style fantasy takes a great deal of work and calculation, but it's one of the most rewarding S&M role-play experiences on the market.

Remember, this is supposed to be *fun*, albeit fun with an edge, so take a reading of your willingness and readiness, jump on the roller coaster, and enjoy the ride!

Getting Down to Business

So you've decided to plan your first "robbery." The hardest thing to do when pulling off a "simulated" burglary is to set a scene that is both

convincing and mindful of the needs of the dominant and the submissive. Since this is a "real time" game and the situation places high
demand on chance, shock, and physicality (not only of the sexual kind),
it's important that things are set in stone so that nobody is pushed farther than s/he can go. On the other hand, the scene also deserves some
"openness" to properly convey the fantasy. It takes a good deal of trust
building, conversation, and planning to bring things to a perfect form
and pitch that both parties can enjoy.

These hints should allow you to set the scene in a way that is safe
and controlled, while still providing room for exploration of the intense
emotions that underlie what is meant to *simulate* a risky situation, fraught
with peril. Note: The following scene can be the cornerstone of fully
fleshed-out role-play scenarios, a template you might adapt to carry
many others.

1. Set the role of the "villain"

As this scene is styled to simulate a real-life strike, your goal is to be
caught off guard in your daily routine, and you play nobody but yourself. This leaves the bulk of the "acting" to be done by the dominant.
The dominant's role will define most of the action in the scenario. If the
dominant is playing a primitive, unskilled burglar, he will use force and
strict bondage to make sure that the hapless homeowner is safely tucked
away while he "raids" the place. Making your intruder a paid thug or
revenge-seeker will allow for an extended period of leisurely domination
and role play. If the dominant and submissive happen to be a sexually
attached couple, he can exercise more predatorily based roles within
the scenario. Any way you look at it, creating a "motive" for the dominant and letting him internalize that driving force will shape the game
to both parties' liking.

2. Set physical restrictions

As your dominant will be coming into this game with the single-minded
goal of subduing and restraining his submissive despite her full resistance,

it is *highly advisable* for you to communicate a detailed list of "things not allowed." This step serves two purposes: (1) a concrete no-no list fixed in the brain should act as a virtual restraining order on both parties, helping perpetrator and victim steer clear of moves that could send things out of control, and (2) foreknowledge of likely action will help you gauge the level of resistance to fit the established limits. If the thrills, for you, lie in the elements of surprise rather than force, yet the fantasy scenario calls for your being fully bound and gagged, your co-conspirator needs to know this so that he can concentrate on the startle aspect and soft-pedal the struggle. If, on the other hand, the force factor is what's going to do it for you, it may be even more important to set limits and spell out specific dos and don'ts. And don't think of moderation as a spoiler—nothing is going to ruin your good time like the unintended consequences of an incidental injury.

3. Set the "damsel's" situation

The dominant himself may have some demands that he would like met. He may wish that you appear in a particular kind of costume and that certain accessories—such useful items as binding materials, duct tape, and bandages—be stocked on the shelves for use during the "ambush." He may want easy access to some personal items and articles of clothing, which may require temporary shifting about of room arrangements. In order for you, the "innocent party," to be blindsided on the night of the heist, it's in your interest to accommodate his vision for "the scene of the crime."

4. Set a time frame

Usually, a loose time frame is set in such games to build tension and maintain focus on the looming element of shock. A given week, or even a month, will be designated for the potential "robbery." A game of cat-and-mouse is played during this period, when your dominant should be studying the patterns of visitors and the hours that you go to work and return. The basic idea is that when the dominant is ready, he can strike at *any time*. This can provide the ultimate sense of shock that often is the biggest thrill in playing a "gotcha" game like this. If you are still somewhat gun-shy, you can set the day and hour in which the game is allowed to happen, and that may work just fine for you. If you are up for more, you can widen the window in which your dom is allowed to pounce. He will be given a set amount of time to plan his attack, and he can spring from any angle he chooses in order to surprise the half-suspecting (or totally unsuspecting) submissive. (For the safety of others, it is best to establish a one-sided email contact in which you may alert the burglar about key times in which visitors are expected and functions are scheduled to happen. This way, you can plan around them without risking a strike "with company." (All you need is a terrified crowd, all 911-ing and bringing down the SWAT team!) This is in consideration of those who will *not* be playing the game. Your dominant partner will not respond to the e-alerts, but he will know key moments in that lying-in-wait period that he best not spring.

5. Set a period of separation

If you've set a specific target date for the break-in, it's a good idea for your dom to absent himself from your life until the big event, as you adjust to the idea of being alone and vulnerable. Don't be tempted to contact the person planning to muscle his way in to "rob" you—during the encounter, you want to be dealing with a stranger, not a lover play-ing a part, so get to work demonizing that bullying desperado! If you've set an extended block of time during which the home invasion can be pulled off—longer than you wish to be split up—at least have him make himself scarce. You want to induce and feed an ominous sense of personal dread, which will add to the impact at the selected moment of "strike."

6. Set the basic role play

Will the dominant be detached, cruel, or forgiving? Will he be asked to wield a weapon? Will he be asked to provide some kind of physical punishment or to say scripted words that the submissive wants to hear? The role-play aspect of this game is central and must be explored. This is not to say that you should script it out entirely, but the submissive should lay out the profile for her "dream captor" so that the dominant can tailor his behavior to fit her needs. The dialogue, the degree of physicality, the props, and other elements should be discussed extensively beforehand to deepen the understanding of what both parties are eager to experience. It's tuning in to the nuances that will enrich your scene, and if you can express the innermost impulses that drew you to role-playing such a scene, the happening will become more richly rewarding for both parties.

7. Set the intruder's entrance into the household

> *The creative act is going from the known to the unknown,*
> *always an anxiety provoking business, The [sic] greater the risk,*
> *the greater the opportunities for disaster, the greater the chance*
> *for an encounter with the wonderful. It's like being a circus*
> *aerialist performing without a net.*
> —DUANE MICHALS, PHOTOGRAPHER[2]

One of the biggest challenges for the dominant in such a game (especially if he's working on an extended time-period fantasy) is gaining entrance to the home, in order to jump and surprise his "prey." After days, or perhaps weeks, of a playful cat-and-mouse game, things take a serious turn at the threshold of your home.

This is risky business—and that's how we like it—but we'd like that circus aerialist to stay airborne! There are many ways to pull off a fake break-in and drive home the fiction of "impending doom," while keeping it pending. Exercising caution is key (you don't want him tackled by a well-meaning neighbor), but beyond that, the challenge is the turn-on from two sides of the equation. This being a robbery fantasy, the house is as much a target as the occupant. In fact, the person may be only peripheral to the scenario being played out and hence treated as such. Gaining forced entry to the house is the first step to binding and gagging the bothersome homeowner, so much attention must be paid here.

HOME INVASION

One tactical plan of attack has the dominant surprising you as you open the door, then forcing his way into the home. This is a common criminal ploy and demonstrates straightaway who's in charge here. It also challenges the dominant because, during that period, the submissive will be on guard and trying to outwit the plotter. Obviously, you're not going to answer the door if you spy the dominant through the peephole and sense "Uh-oh, tonight's the night!" Diversionary tactics may be needed to offset such warning signals. He might even resort to subterfuge, calling ahead to say he'd like to stop by, for instance, keeping it casual, and then springing into action on his main mission. By whatever means he chooses to force his way through the front door, the action is going to spark alarm and startle you into submission within the role-play scene the two of you have devised.

KEY TRADE

If you live in an urban area where the population is on high alert, or even a suburban community where neighbors actually know and watch out for one another, it may be wise to let the dominant have a key, so as not to set alarm bells jangling among the snoopy set. If, to your mind, this threatens the overlay of "realism," one can fudge the rules by letting him "steal" a key along the way, so that your intruder appears to have mastered the lock-picking skills of any decent crook. As your dominant is presumably not a career criminal, this must be one of the scene-setting tricks on which the two of you are in collusion.

WINDOWS

Leaving a ground-floor window unlocked, even open, at all times is another good strategy, challenging the dominant to sneak in unobserved, day or night. It also allows him access to scope out your living quarters even before the "attack."

FULL BREAK-IN

If you live in a secluded area, or simply are willing to have your dominant stage a full-scale break-in for the sake of arch reality, you might actually grant him license to cause minor damage (a busted window latch, for instance) by smashing his way into the apartment/home. We all know what a break-in can entail, and while such a scene can be exciting, neither Mr. H nor I normally would suggest something this rash. That said, if the full break-in appeals to you, we do so with a caution: Specify property damage limits, and stress the word *property*— precautions must be taken to avoid any collateral physical harm to either party. And a disclaimer—RISKY BUSINESS! You've been warned.

Other Scenarios

The strategizing elements in the robbery scene play may be amended to fit many other kinds of scenes. While the plot details will differ, many of the technical details may be appropriated. Below, in lieu of an "Exercises" section for this chapter, I will cover theatrical, nontechnical aspects of other appealing scenarios to fire up your imagination about possibilities for new scenes.

The Female Soldier/Spy War Captive

WHAT: You are the notorious spy, a prize "get," now at the mercy of your merciless antagonist, who means to have a hanky-panky good time with you before handing you over to the authorities.

WHEN: As this is a martial fantasy, the time of day isn't important as long as it's on military time. The spy faces the firing squad at 0600 hours, giving your ruthless captor a whole night to get what he wants out of you.

HOW: Well, the two most dreaded fates to befall a captured soldier or spy would be to suffer interrogation as a bound and helpless prisoner or to be held in the field at the mercy of an unscrupulous enemy combatant. Buy or improvise some military uniforms. Clear out an area of your living space to create a nice sparse setting to serve as a barracks or, perhaps, a bare-bones interrogation room. Look into military code words and protocols to set up the scene.

WHY: She's the *enemy* of course! She deserves punishment! What could hold richer promise than enemy territory for the setting of a scene of dominance and submission?

The Stripper/Call Girl (Objectification)

WHAT: Your role model—*BUtterfield 8* call girl or Parisian streetwalker—will determine your wardrobe. It will be Park Avenue at the high end or red-light district at the low. Going all out, in either direction, builds attraction.

WHEN: The illusion of secrecy is a grand addition to a scene like this. The night belongs to these ladies of the night, and the best time of night is late nite, when the seedy hotel is at peak turnover and the staff of the gentlemen's club isn't looking anyway. Remember, you are creating the illusion of carrying out an illegal act in which you are being hired to fulfill a man's every desire. This won't be a public scene. Use everything you can dream up to amplify the feeling of an illicit moment.

HOW: Set it up via phone call and email. Use a fake name for the exchange and choose a private place to meet and be entertained. The more you can do to create the illusion that you are doing something secretive and illicit, the easier you will find it to slip into your characters. Both the shameless hooker with the exposed flesh and the come-hither stare and the high-class hooker in the cocktail dress look to their Johns for upkeep, and both expect to sexily shed their costumes for a price.

WHY: Many men fantasize about paying a sex partner, in order to be completely in control of her, and, as well, many women fantasize about being the object of that interaction. Exercising this form of power declares the sexual encounter impersonal and encourages the woman to push herself to please the man, in hopes of fulfilling his desires, which she may or may not share. It's the fantasy of the debased woman, representing "paid-for goods," that encourages a man to engage the animal instincts of his nature, to feel justified in making "indecent" demands. Likewise, imagining yourself in the position of chattel should release you from the natural compunctions, allowing you to allow him to "get what he paid for."

The Lady in Debt to a Loan Shark, Mobster, or Criminal Tough Guy

WHAT: It's time to pay the bad man! This fantasy is built on the familiar story of the desperate soul in debt to the loan shark who now faces a thug sent over to collect money. As the story goes, not having the money means that a "price" must be extracted, encouraging the debtor to make good on future payments. Of course, as your scene plays out, the price will result in your being dominated, humiliated, and taught a lesson in hard finances!

WHEN: Since this is a "criminal drop-in," it should happen late at night. Keep the atmosphere raw, should you decide to throw in a little cat-and-mouse hunt action on the streets as he follows you home. Just remember, this is a scene where the drama is meant to create an edge to make the moment of impact explosive and *muy* uncomfortable.

HOW: The dress and timing won't matter as much as the ambience. Create an atmosphere of agonizing worry and threat and turn that into the theme of the show. This is a chance for the dom to be more physical than usual and to use a coarser tone in his verbal exchanges. He is here not only to teach you a lesson but also to get his money's worth for the amount that you owe him! This is the time for your partner to play tough. As with the robbery fantasy, you can co-opt movieland criminal elements and methods to play out the scene. The rough language and behavior of intimidation are encouraged. Having your head yanked back by your ponytail while cruel threats are whispered into your ear may be just what you need to nail your own great performance.

WHY: For the same reason Brando and De Niro, Depp and Pacino, and all the rest of Hollywood's A-listers lust after the tough-guy roles— getting to act the sexy badass, siding with the mobsters and molls, wiseguys and goodfellas, can be such good racy *un*wholesome fun!

The Escaped Convict

WHAT: Think *Cape Fear* c. 1962 or 1991. The escaped convict needs a place to hide and some, shall we say, amusing diversion. Are you prepared to be that entertainment? This closely mirrors the burglary scene, as it works from the forced-entry plot point and is a high-melodrama scenario. His needs and your needs might be the same but it is *certain* that he is going to take advantage of your home and everything you own.

WHEN: Anytime. A desperate criminal isn't going to bend to *your* schedule to break in and take control. You can play it several ways: He can simply break in, at any time, day or night; he can lie in wait for you as you return from work, springing from the bushes to catch you off guard; or he can follow you home after a shopping trip or drinks with the girls.

HOW: Bondage plays a huge part in this escapade as the desperate villain has grave (!) reasons to prevent you from alerting the authorities during his visit to your humble home. Use bondage, have him move the scene at a slow pace to draw out the torment, and script the interactions to work via manipulation on the part of both characters. This can be an extended, long-play scene that gives you a lot of procedural range. You might have him leave you bound and helpless while he uses your phone or watches television in between sessions of using you for his own purposes. A prison uniform is a great asset, but short of that, go for the run-down criminal look. (Hint: An orange jumpsuit should do it . . . when's the last time you saw a convict wearing stripes?) Your captor is supposed to be a rough 'n' ready man with a desperate streak, so play that up in the scene. Have your lover not shave for a little while. Think outside the houseboat on this one . . .

WHY: Desperation, thy name is Escaped Convict. What a mouth-watering temptation to take on the persona of the guy with nothing to lose. Psychologically, emotionally, "owning" these roles—the heartless villain to your innocent dame—has to be the ultimate turn-on for a dom. Work it!

The Punishment

WHAT: Whatever your lover wants! You are allowing him to extract payback for your crimes, so you will dress as he wishes, do and say what he wants. In short, you are his slave for the night and will do exactly as he says in order to earn his forgiveness. You might be made to wear or say something embarrassing and you *will* agree, just to remain in his good graces!

WHEN: Whenever *he* wants! You are on *his* time frame and you will do as commanded when you are commanded! Part of the fun is not knowing what he will want or when, but it's *your* debt. PAY UP!

HOW: However *he* wants it! Enacting the paying-off-your-debt scene comes at the cost of your becoming a total love slave for him. This is where he can get creative, subjecting you to all sorts of tests that will turn you both on while pushing your limits. Unlike other scenes, this isn't about creating the illusion of force but, rather, your choosing to work off debts, so play up the choice angle and show a little resistance. Negotiate, but keep in mind that it's his way or, now that you've fessed up to a lifetime of little sins, a near future filled with tons of tension and no absolution. Your call now; his . . . forever after?

WHY: Everyone has had a partner hurt his or her feelings—something done or said that was mean or hurtful, e.g., charging excessively on your joint credit card (oh, naughty!), interrupting an important moment, and otherwise making life miserable in some way. Exacting revenge—"returning the favor"—is an irresistible element for use in role play. While your relationship may be power-neutral day to day, with gripes accruing on both sides of the partnership, it will profit the dominant/submissive gamesmanship if you dredge up your *own* indiscretions and toss them out as punishment-worthy. This will invite your partner to demand various acts of submission as payback for your misdeeds. It's much like the "No-Scenario" scenario (see below), fueled in this case by specific "sins" and the resultant grudges.

The "No-Scenario" Scenario

WHAT: Whatever you want! Since you are not following a "scene" plan, you can wear what you want and say what you want—and he can spank what he wants! This kind of interaction really isn't a scene so much as free play, based on a collaboration of actions. Since you are not indulging a full-blown fantasy with clearly defined character roles, the world opens to spontaneous play with improvised props and plot drivers.

WHEN: When are you free?

HOW: However you like! You are "in the moment," as they say in the acting biz, so let the moment dictate your desires and pleasures.

WHY: Because you want to. This is traditional dominance and submission at its core. It's an example of what can happen when you just want a spot at the bottom while you hand him complete control. There is no gimmick, other than the need to give up a little control in return for an evening of pleasure.

A Cheat Sheet on Setting Limits as You Script Your Role-Play Scene

You may wish to tuck this concise slate of notes into your scripting folder and use as a quick-reference checklist. For a full discussion of the importance and setting of limits in DSRP, see chapter 2.

1. Lay out the pace and level of force you wish your partner to use in his physical actions—slow, gentle, harsh, fast and frightening, etc.

2. Let him know if verbal humiliation play is in or out of bounds. Get specific, e.g., *bitch* is okay but *slut* is not—you get the picture.

3. Tell him which physical faux punishments do and do not appeal, and set boundaries accordingly. If you wish only verbal taunts and no physical discipline, say so. Further, let him know if restraints are to be allowed and, if so, which ones. For instance: gags and cuffs, yes; tying up, no.

4. Do tell or remind him what you like sexually and what you won't go for, to ensure he doesn't equate DRSP with a free-for-all. ("Oh boy, I get to f*** you up the . . ." "Huhh? Slow down, skippy, no you do not!")

5. What tone of voice do you wish him to use? Firm? Gentle but firm? Forceful? Aggressive? Calm and authoritative? You'll want to specify this because in DSRP, as in all personal interactions, tone of voice modulates behavior. Better yet, send him a YouTube clip of a movie scene in which you like the demeanor, tone, and style of a suitably imposing male actor. I list BDSM movies in the appendix, if you'd like to check out the male dominants and find a model that suits your fancy.

Once you've resolved the details of these important details—the shaping of character to script, that is—then think about how best to instruct your player. To keep it friendly, I recommend it be over a glass of wine at a chichi restaurant (with well-spaced tables), keeping it festive and more formal than a bossy lecture across the kitchen table. I find that if I have to bring up something I find "difficult" to my lover, I'm more comfortable spilling outside the home front. Kinky talk is easier and sweeter in a dreamy locale removed from everyday life and the distractions of the attention-hogging dog. Just a suggestion . . .

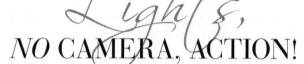

NO CAMERA, ACTION!

THE NITTY-GRITTY OF STAGING A DSRP SCENE: COSTUMES,
SET DESIGN, MOOD-ENHANCING PROPS, AND EFFECTS

chapter eight

*"Nobody told us anything about the facts of life. We were all ignorant,
and if we had known we'd have thought it disgusting. Certainly, I and all
my close friends would have considered ourselves defiled if we hadn't come to
marriage as virgins . . . At deb dances there were a few girls of whom
we'd say 'They do it, you know!'—though perhaps all they did was cuddle
and kiss behind bushes. But even that was definitely disapproved of. . . .
If boys tried to pounce, the word soon got around. They were described as
NSIT—not safe in taxis—and girls warned each other to avoid them."*

—BRITISH DEBUTANTE WHO "DID THE SEASON"
IN 1938 LONDON[1]

*"TaxiTreat's Condom Vending Machines May Hit
NYC Cabs This Summer, CEO Says"[2]*
—HEADLINE, *HUFFINGTON POST*

Whoa! Reading those zeitgeisty tea leaves from the backseat of a
1930s taxicab, may we celebrants of sexual freedom not toast the
fact that in just two generations of cultural evolution, our Love Laws

have taken a postmodern turn off the tsk-tsk path toward the let's-get-real-already? The focus of Mommy's Safety First Lecture to Daughter has shifted from preserving virginity to protecting health/preventing unwanted pregnancy—from "no sex (before marriage)" to "safe sex."

So-o-o-o twentieth century, all that fussing over social convention, prioritizing propriety over pleasure. Poor little lambs, our carefully reared sisters, looking for counsel in all the wrong places. And here *we* are—the Gen Xers, Yers, and beyond—ruled by the Safe Sex imperative and, it appears, soon to be able to exercise it from the backseat of a . . . *taxicab! Openly* flirting with the romantic notion of fantasy role play, designing the scenes, costuming the players, *enjoying* the adventure. What say I dedicate one special scene to the deb class of '38, their randy-tagged escorts, and, to be charitable, their well-meaning mothers? I'm thinking perhaps a reprise of the naughty modern Brit Kate Winslet in *Revolutionary Road*, being mounted in the front seat of a guy's Cadillac. Or, in literal adherence to the taxi theme, how about the hot sex in a cab in the 1980 erotic crime thriller *Dressed to Kill* (Angie Dickinson is *something*; rent it!)

In Defense of Carpe Diem and . . . Going for It

Costuming is all important to any theatrical production, and staging for DSRP is no different. In this, I was programmed to be a hopeless loser in the Scene Stakes. I hate dressing up, all the frills, twirls, and girly jingle-bell theatrics. So much energy and commitment. Nails (both sets), hot irons, surgically straight eyeliner streaks, scenting, buffing, and those pinchy heels—frankly, missy, I never had the patience. It just all seemed so exhausting and a smidge cheesy. And furthermore, rather pointless, as I had chosen to live in an unconventional, some may say outré, world that didn't demand such fuss. Until, that is, I was muscled into it by Mr. H (Mr. H?! My unpretentious artist Mr. H? To borrow an utterly adorable oldie locution, "Who'd a thunk it?") He would spell out all his *très* specific femmy dress fantasies, and I would flicker a pish-pish of an eye roll. We were at a standstill. I had no desire to be all gussied up and trotted out like a star pony to satisfy his visual fancy. I'm a lazy kitty.

But Jesus God, he kept harping on "the look"—his ideal look, that is—for role play. What he wanted: classic, high-end black lingerie; a smart, tailored business shirt and suit; the "geisha gone to London" makeup and glassy-shine hair slicked back into a bun, *à la* Robert Palmer's iconic "Addicted to Love" video. In other words, a fierce and sexy Bitch Means Business (flattering, because that was my adopted nine-to-five MO, though I slothfully refused to dress the part).

I'd snap back: "Will you stop with the dressing-up shit? You're like obsessed with women's clothing. No bleed'n man I know cares about styles of lingerie or dress. They'd hardly notice if a supermodel was in Daisy Buchanan ethereal, Daisy Dukes, or Bond girl brut-glam. What's wrong with you?!"

"Not true," says he.

Hmmm, interesting. Okay, I'm listening. Mr. H busts out the goods and explains himself: "Every man has very specific tastes in women's, particularly *his* woman's, dress and lingerie styles."

I can't believe this. "*What?* Like, who? How many men have told you this? And don't include your weirdo arty friends."

He responds: "*Everyone.* My artist friends, businessman friends, a professor chum at Columbia University, my union chief, and guys on his construction crew."

The whole mélange of men at any given salty beerhouse bro bar in the city, it sounds like. Wow. Okay, so why don't men tell women exactly what style of clothes and lingerie they like and would like to see on them, huh?

"Because fashion is not their lingo," he says.

All right. So how specific are their tastes?

"Very. As specific as yours."

I suppose they just feel uncomfortable expressing their clothing preferences and desires, probably afraid we will find it strange that they care as much as chicks do? So they're stuck with "Yes, dear, that's hot," as they fantasize a completely different look they've seen in a Victoria's Secret online ad? Poor little monkeys. Well, jeez Louise, if fashion means so much to you guys, in gearing up for the main event, fine, tell me exactly what you want me to wear.

Mr. H tosses off specifics like it's been his secret Christmas wish list for years. Damn if the boy doesn't know precisely what he wants in his playroom:

1. A pinstripe pencil skirt a tad above the knees.

2. An expensive white business shirt and swank blazer.

3. Hair in a bun.

4. Medium-height heels, black.

5. Nude stockings.

6. Posh, understated black silk lingerie that looks more functional than frilly.

This, it surfaced, was his shopping list for our DSRP scene.

Hemming, hawing, I slapped on a pair of jeans and Uggs with a serviceable L.L. Bean ski jacket, no makeup, hair a not-hot mess, and trudged through the sidewalk slush to Barney's,[3] a chichi chic department store in Manhattan where absolutely *everyone*, the counter girls included, is more fabulous than you. Took one last puff on my ciggy, stomped on it with my clodhopper boots, and, like an unwelcome bull in a snotty china shop, I busted through the revolving starlet doors like I was heaving a stalled car up the road. This type of place yawns me to death—got over it when I was seventeen.

Well-l-l, I was wrong! It was a hopping good time. Fun, fun, fun. Cursing under my breath—"I have no time for this nonsense, I own enough formal clothing, this is a waste of my hard-won dollars," y'know, "adult, sensible thoughts"—I found myself in a sexy candy land of polished glass. My eyes would sneak a girly peek at some hot little dress or stockings with a burlesque naughty seam up the back of the leg. Sparkly eye shadows in tropical island fish-scale shades and Marilyn Monroe pink-puff lip glosses that whispered, "Y'mmm, please tell the gentleman I accept his invitation." A sexy police line-up of sleek little outlaw high heels, all so glam and femme fatale danger-ous. The sparsely positioned silver hangers wearing Barbara Stanwyck sharp-shoulder cut blazers. I was getting glitz butterfly jolts of giddi-ness in this surprisingly seductive effort to please my man and satisfy his lust for DSRP with a glammed-up me. Yes, I had to admit I was having a lot of old-fashioned fun, damn it. Like a caviar treat, it sud-denly came to me, as I recalled the words of Marilyn Monroe in her last interview: "Fame is like caviar. It's good to have caviar, but not every damned day," followed by childlike giggles.

My madcap take for the day (the prices were ghastly! breathtak-ing!): (1) Marie Antoinette–grade mascara and (2) not just any old big shot's white shirt but a Qatar Airways business class white shirt. So, the trip to Barney's served its purpose—it got me thinking girlier where it counts (in my romantic life and among my female pack) and earned me an admiring low whistle from Mr. H on the shirt (good thing—I think I'm still paying it off).

I needed this treat of transformation, from girl slopping it up on the couch watching TV with Mr. H to a thoughtfully manufactured hot property. As it turned out, the effort was a vital buildup to a sur-prise DSRP scene. Just days before, I had been hanging with Mr. H, comfortable in looking like "Sadie married lady" crap in shabby paja-mas and scarfing down takeout pizza, overweight (a good ten pounds, owing to the stress of running my film business), my face broken out from menstrual-ness. I playfully said to Mr. H, "Tsss, I'm fat and covered with zits, whatever . . . " He cute-kissed and affectionately played along, bap-tizing me Zit Pig. I busted a gut laughing and threw myself on top of him. "Zit Pig demands sex right now or Zit Pig is going to eat you. Aarrr!" Faint pleading cries of "nooo, nooo" from him. Cute, but how the hell was Zit Pig supposed to get in the mood and, even harder, get present-able for a caviar treat of delicious DSRP? I had to de-hausfrau and zap into being a new mystery woman of our fantasies, if we were to be Movie Stars Meeting for the First Time on the Set of a Romantic Film.

No way around it, I told myself. You must do the starlet dressing and create the set. Otherwise I'm scruffy little Zit Pig and he's scruffy Teddy the Couch Bear. And I pull from experience when I say that the more work you put into costuming for your movie set, the more fame-caviar lust rush you shall have to devour. It may seem a bit overkill and stagey, but it works! And I highly recommend that you and your partner rent a hotel or motel room at least once and really go for the film-set feel for your dominant/submissive scene. It can turn you and your play from Norma-Not-Meatloaf-Again!-Jean to Marilyn-Caviar-Monroe. Nothing like a caper on foreign soil to ratchet up the kink meter! Read on.

A Confessional Tale and a Prologue to Your Own Production

Let me spotlight my claim to dreamiest DSRP fame, an impromptu adventure that developed from an out-of-this-world opportunity. Mr. H accompanied me on a business trip to La La Land for a fetish film shoot. It was to be staged on location at a five-star Beverly Hills hotel, where, H'wood legend has it, Liz Taylor used to book rooms for incognito recovery after facelift surgeries. It was a *crème de la crème* haunt, which I picked for its singularly luxurious-looking rooms. It was also to be our Hollywood crash pad for what turned into a business/pleasure trip of glorious, unabashed decadence. And why not?

We had two shoots. The first was with a submissive, a beautiful African American film student and cool Cali artist kid who loved being in femdom videos (masked to hide his identity). I had booked early, oblivious to the fact that our stay was to coincide with Academy Awards weekend, so the snazzy hotel was supernaturally sugar-frosted with celebs and the attendant paparazzi, who parked themselves outside hoping to snap a long-lens hot cover shot of some celeb shenanigans through the hotel room balconies.

Scene: we have a gorgeous young black man (a UCLA film student who fancies being dominated by women) standing on the bed, hands tied to the sliding custom-crafted wood doors above the headboard, waiting to be domme-whipped. The bed is in direct view of the balcony and beyond, which means that the paparazzi pack swarming the Beverly Hills sidewalk . . . *shit shit shit!* I run to the balcony to lower the shades and spot a photographer putz staring up at our scene, dumbfounded and frozen as if in shock, giving him pause—thank God!—before lifting his camera. "Shut it down!" I freak. "OMG, he's going to like send the picture to the hotel and we'll be like kicked out or, worse, sued for filming in here!" Mr. H tries to calm me down, but I'm in a dervish whirl of anxiety and panic. I call to ask room service if they have chocolate-covered strawberries on the menu, a good-night treat after a stressful day. They don't but, ever agreeable, they offer to do a custom dip for me. I also ask for an ashtray and matches, even though we both know the room is designated nonsmoking, and, without comment, they send up the contraband. The matches imprinted with the hotel's logo are delivered like little treasures, in a mini-mini Ralph Lauren–looking bag with braided silk handles, a presentation worthy of a room-service Hope Diamond. Ridiculous. We laugh. But I can see why La Mama Bear Liz found the joint so just-right. It's a movie-star mirage come to life.

Cut to: the next day. I jolt out of my five-star cloud bed and get straight to work, hightailing it to the L.A. pro rental shop for more filming lights, as ours have blown. We're in high gear, readying the set for the beautiful Jessica Jaymes, a famous, high-end adult film star, a former ballerina, and one of the most gorgeous women I've ever laid eyes on. She arrives, and we start the scene. She's wearing a vintage black Chanel suit and a blond wig. The scripted scene is that she's picked up a businessman in the hotel bar. We sneak into the hotel hallway and, like thieves, steal a shot of her leading the sub/actor/businessman to our room. She gently presses her claws into his chest and coaxes him onto the puff bed. Seductively ties his hands to the decorative sliding doors above, pulls off the blond wig to expose her glossy, long, dark hair, and then, in a smoky-smooth voice, says, "What, you thought you picked up a dumb blond?" She gives a sultry, sneering, half "gotcha" laugh and turns the tables, teasing him sexually and dominating him as he lies helplessly trussed. I have my stunning star slip into the pearl oval bathtub and slither around in the bubbles, just for burlesque, S&M'y kicks. I grab a bottle of Veuve Clicquot from the minibar and tell her to pour it over her ballerina-perfect body and exquisite round breasts. Drawing from her professional past as a classically trained dancer, she puts on a froth of a siren seafoam dance that would make sailors and sea gods lose their minds. The sub actor remains tied up, now watching her from the "penalty box," a shower stall facing her lagoon bath and raining frigid water onto his naked body. She leads him, hands bound, out of the shower and proceeds to talk tough, demanding that he perform sensual acts to her bidding with threats of blackmailing him, like a good femme fatale. After thus forcing him to pleasure her, the villainous vixen instructs him to serve as her boudoir stool as she gets dressed, touches up her makeup, and re-dons the wig. All the while, she's staring into a mirror encircled by warm, red-yellow globe light bulbs, adding a touch of the old Hollywood pizzazz. Then out he goes.

Awww, rats! The stressful but steamy shoot is over! After the actors depart, I flop on the bed. Mr. H, having shot the scene, is in the mood. He has a plan. Well, we have the costumes of his waking dreams— executive-chic business suit, stockings, and heels from Jessica's wardrobe; the actor's ties and extra stockings for bondage; the dreamy swank hotel room. He suggests, or rather, he *informs* me, that we are to use the rudiments of the scene I created but in reverse roles. I am to be the sub and he will be turning the tables and domming *moi. C'est fantastique.* Normally I would scoff at such an elaborate set-up, with all its pomp and frilly circumstance, but now I give it a *Gone with the Wind* twirl.

Mr. H tells me to get dressed in my star costume and meet him in the hotel bar downstairs in twenty-five minutes—on the dot, or I'll have to "pay," i.e., be punished later. He vanishes. I light a cig and illicitly (and thoughtlessly) leave it burning on the side of the expensive wood makeup table. Preparation feels like a chore at first but then I get into it, playacting a starlet getting ready for the Academy Awards (and fantasizing about *my* reward!). My twenty-five minutes is nearly up when I notice that my spent cig has burned down, leaving a tar-black scar branded into the handsome wood tabletop. Fuck fuck fuck. Okay, so the management was right to declare the suite off limits to smokers, with careless brats like me roaming the premises. I'm imagining my bill . . . what? an extra $3k for the table? Way to bust the shoot budget, Alexis!

A ball of curse words, and on my last nerve, I head to the bar. I step into the elevator and there stands a bigass six-foot-something mega-famous movie star with a couple of annoying hangers-on. We lock eyes and—shit! Now I'm even more unraveled.

I slip into the swanky, candlelit bar and feel Mr. H come up behind me, grabbing my inner thigh. "Looking to pick up a movie star? Follow me up to my room or I'll tell the concierge what you've been up to in there." I know he means the illegal smoking, filming, etc. "Walk closely behind me," he says. We are alone in the elevator and he commandingly whips me around and presses me up against the wall, slips his hand up my Chanel suit jacket, and pinches my nipple. "Oaaahh," I moan. "I'll release it if you promise to get into the bed and spread your legs and arms while I tie you up and stuff your panties in your mouth. No? Then we'll have a talk with the concierge and you'll have to explain why you were being a very bad girl and a slut in their hotel." I know he won't do this, but still, all he has to do is dial nine on the hotel phone to cause me to scream. I don't want to test how close to doomsday he's willing to go.

Ding! Our floor. I walk with haughty attitude into the room and assume his dictated position. As he's tying me up—normally I'd be wailing like a banshee, complaining that the bondage gear is too tight—I sense something surreal in the luxurious atmosphere of our fantasy set that allows me to escape the membrane of real and flee into Neverland. Shedding the shackles of Zit Pig, I'm thrust into a starring role that simply wouldn't have played out in my couchy-homey, frumped-up digs in New York. I'm allowed sips of Champagne and puffs of his cigarette in exchange for giving him "sexy favors" and allowing him—for the very first time—to hogtie me, using my stockings and his tie. Oddly, I don't suffer the claustrophobic desperation that's always accompanied such bondage activity. Rather, I'm swept up into the "movie"—Alexis releasing her inner Monroe.

While I'm languishing in a humiliating hog-tie, Mr. H leisurely teases me for at least an hour. I'm helpless yet overflowing with arousing impulses. He unties my legs and gently grabs my hair, leading me at a crawl into the pearly bathtub, which he's filled. He sets up a chair and commands me to do a Jessica Jaymes sexy tease for him. Zit Pig doing a Dita Von Teese Salome number? You must be . . . I say, "No no no," and turn red and laugh out loud. He slaps me and repeats the threat to dial nine, then calls me a badly behaved, dirty-rotten, spoiled little girl. I sink into the heat of the tub, and he commands me to masturbate. I protest but comply, and my embarrassment fades as I relish his own discomfort in trying to hide the signs of his arousal. He stays in character, cold. His self-control makes me hotter.

He hands me a towel and orders me to mop up all the bubbles that my Dita Von Teesing has caused to spill over onto the marble floor. He stands over me in his suit, arms crossed, making sure I do a proper cleanup, like a well-trained scullery maid. "This will teach you to respect the rules and not to trash hotel rooms like a selfish, slutty starlet." I do feel like a slutty, spoiled twit for burning the beautiful wood. I decide to tell him what I did. He puffs up his chest in anger and disapproval, raises an eyebrow, bends me over the makeup table, and spanks me hard. Locks me in the walk-in closet for twenty minutes, while he lectures me through the door. I beg to be let out. He says yes, under one condition: I am to remain on all fours, wearing a panty gag, while he has his way with me. Then I'm to suffer certain "cosmetic indignities" for being a spoiled and thoughtless girl, with no regard or respect for the generous hotel staff, carelessly burning up the furniture, leaving chocolate-strawberry smears all over the bed sheets. I allow him his wish, and my guilt is assuaged by the deprecating feelings Mr. H engenders through insults and enslaving. I begin to feel gentle and receptive, more malleable actress than tyrannical director, and I'm not unhappy to discover that within me there's room for the yin and yang elements of both. I melt into a vulnerable and open Monroe and my sexuality supersedes my anxiety.

Afterward, Mr. H scrubs and buffs me up with lavender sweet soap and a bridal-white, preposterously fluffy hotel towel. We call room service and order a bunch of appetizers, one being—just had to do it—caviar. It arrives on the proper glass plate, atop shaved ice, with the proper compartments for the proper tidbits that caviar demands: the egg yolks delicately separated from the minced egg whites, crème fraîche, toast points, and yes, little mother-of-pearl spoons (imagine Peter the Great allowing the taste of his fish eggs to be tainted by a silver spoon—zounds!). Suddenly very posh and in control, I tell Mr. H to watch as I pretend to do something truly degenerate and unruly, mashing the eggs yokes with the egg whites together. *Arrrr!* Oh, the horror! Truly, the caviar is divine and the perfect topping to my absurdly decadent role-play experience as a sub. The scene has been, at once, everything I detest and . . . the most delicious sexual experience I have ever had. Puff puff tee hees, dahhlings.

If you can't swing a five-star hotel and Champagne baths with beluga, don't fret. Borrowing from the thrifty prop master's handbook, I have some artful tips on how to turn living and workspace into play space—call it your own private Shrine to Hedonism.

Before we roll camera, let's plan the film scene. First a checklist and then details.

The DSRP producer's checklist:

1. Costumes

2. Location and set design

3. Enhancements: music, scents, mood lighting, maybe?

Costumes

Do you have in mind a fantasy costume suited to a particular persona? It can be as real-world simple as a striking cocktail dress or frilly negligee—perhaps a treasured piece you've been saving for a special occasion—or as Hollywood as a sexy French maid, a dutiful secretary, a Persian princess, a disheveled captive straight out of a shipwreck film, a *Pretty Woman* call girl, a shy schoolgirl, or Catwoman. Mine your memory to recall a film character you found titillating and work her into your DRSP scene. Or break out your private erotic story and imagine what that female sub character would be wearing. If this feels more chore than amusement, ask your lover what costume or attire he imagines it might fun to play with. That approach, in fact, might be best, as soliciting his input serves dual purposes: By actively seeking to please him, you're easing yourself into the sub role, and by playing to his stated fantasy wishes, you're assured a *warm* reception. Building up excitement through anticipation is a great gambit, with each of you feeding into the other's desire—works like surefire virtual foreplay!

Do you have a character you'd like him to role-play? Again, read over your erotic story and, if you haven't already detailed his description, imagine what your fantasy dominant might be wearing. Choose an arousing character—charmer or villain—from a favorite film or a novel, recall his attributes, his style, then decide if the casting will work with your own choice of sub character in your role-play scenario. Is he Christian Grey in a powerhouse business suit, a strict soldier or policeman (so easy to fall for a uniform!), a thief/burglar, a boss figure, a stable boy, a manly peasant worker with rough hands, a sadistic schoolmaster, a John who hires you for sex, a disdainful royal prince, your surly pimp, a cowboy who knows how to control and train his filly, a lecherous stepfather *(oh, my!* and *oooo la la!)*? Dive in and drag the naughty out! If you decide to dress up your man, you needn't go all Halloween-y. Maybe jeans and a T-shirt for the union worker, a pair of manly boots and a scary thick leather belt for the soldier, a pair of cuffs for the policeman, a slick suit for the boss. And if this all seems too much prep work for you, or you sense it may be too embarrassing for him, no worries. As I see it, *your* costume should carry the scene. You're the sub/star, the object of a shared fantasy, and he's the pawn, working for you. Too, most men need the 3-D visual, whereas we're famous for being able to visual-*ize*, a superior talent, no?

Ask your lover which lingerie styles turn him on. If he clams up and gives an OMG-what-does-she-really-want-from-me look, help him out. Pull up a lingerie website—Agent Provocateur is a good one, though pricey, for posh-sexy—and flip through the screens, having him point out which looks grab him. (If you watch his face, you won't need his words, and I warn you, his reactions may be a *big* surprise). This will give you a head start in fishing out his dream fantasy role-play girl. If he chooses the daisy'd camisole, that's a hot tip that his fantasies probably run to the soft, virginal damsel. If he points to the slick black lingerie, he may prefer a challenging, dominant-type fantasy girl. If he goes for the burlesque, his fantasy might call for a racy sexpot he can spank for being "naughty." It's safe to say that the attire he responds to reveals his sexual fantasy femmes.

My friends and I have played this game, and I can tell you that couples generally agree on lingerie style preferences. No surprise here, as our fashion tastes reflect our personas, and our lovers are attracted to us because they like what they see. If his preferences align with yours, yet your lingerie drawer these days runs to dingy gray pieces picked up at last year's street fair, well, you've gotten lazy and complacent, and this fantasy exercise may spur a shopping binge. If, however, he gloms on to the virginal daisy-chain pastel prints when your wardrobe runs to boyish, bossypants black, uhhh, you might need to rethink your choice not in undies but in guys. Eeek. Is he *really* that into the *true* you? The lingerie test. Silly? Hmmm, maybe so, maybe not. Best raise your antennae.

Location and Set Design

Remember, form follows function. Here are some ideas for titillating places that may inspire your inner voluptuary.

For indoor private:

Think about splurging on a swanky hotel room for the night, but if that's a budget-busting idea, even a Motel 6 can be made to work. Raw and seedy is just the ticket if, let's say, you're to play an upper-crust lady of the *haut monde*, taken hostage by a rough-and-tumble man who hauls you to an out-of-the-way motel knowing that no one is likely to notice if you scream. Tasty! If either idea is out of the question, then get creative with your apartment or a room in your house. Dress it up or down. Flickering firelight can romanticize any space, so it's light up the candles and off with the overheads and table lamps. You're a harem sex slave? Hang sheets on the windows and over the furniture. With the lights out, you'll feel like you're in a Moroccan kasbah. Didn't you do this as a kid? Gussy up your room to look like the royal princess quarters of the castle? Build a bunker in your army fort?

This is adult play, and it will serve the present pursuit to unleash those wild imaginings of your childhood and the wilder escapades of your rakish young adulthood. Put on your favorite disco song—"Hot Shot," circa 1978, by Karen Young (a fave in underground seventies gay clubs), is a great one—and get shak'n, moving, dancing . . . decorating the pad while you groove out to the celebrated sounds of—no other word for it—*freedom*! Talk about creative license! Haven't we all salivated in recalling, or listening to, the deliciously racy tales of the roaring seventies and eighties when Andy and Edie and Truman and Cher and Bianca (and, and, and . . .) acted and dressed and carried on as they damn well pleased? When disco dancers, fashion- and art-world scenesters, and other self-created characters knocked themselves out competing in the original costume sweeps? When the glam de la glam Studio 54, the club that put disco on the map, showed the whole world how to throw a party—done up like a harem one night and a barnyard with haystacks the next. I say turn back the clock! Take inspiration from the event planner who dumped four tons (!) of glitter on 54's dance floor one New Year's Eve—it was like "standing on stardust," the owner said. So, unless you're introducing mousy Miss Goody Girl Scout on opening night, cue the arty of all parties and you'll come up with your own ideas for a *scaled-down* bacchanalia (seriously, no one wants to be picking glitter out of her panties months later, as the revelers at the glitterfest were said to have done).

For country outdoors:

Camping offers a great instant portal to fantasy land. Even a backyard will do. On some starry, starry night, who better than Tarzan to fire-strip Jane's social conditioning and spark those primal responses? Natural settings work well for hostage scenes, a meeting with your lonely soldier boy in the fort, a playdate with the rough, tough lumberjack, or an encounter with the wild-man forest beast—you get the picture.

For the adventurous types: Antsy anticipation and tightrope walking breed loads of excitement. Have your dominant character pick you up on the side of a lonely road at night. Did your car break down? Of course it did. Blush. "Oh, who is this handsome guy pulling over to save me? Uh oh, might he hold me captive? Do I owe him a 'favor' for picking me up? Haha, little does he know that I faked my car crisis! I'm a sexpot hooker and I've just trapped a hot John to pleasure—and my 'favors' are price-tagged!" All right, this is one of my pop-up fantasies. I just went for it. What's yours?

For city outdoors:

Bustling city streets. Who's up for a cat-and-mouse game? Meet your lover at a coffee shop/bar/restaurant and don't speak. The plan is that he follows you out and through the streets until he finds an alleyway, with the coast clear, to grab and threaten you before strong-arming you back to your apartment. Then start playing! Another winning scene: Go out for a dressy dinner and have him fondle you and firmly grab your hands in a lock position under the table. He tells you what he's going to do to you once you're home. You are mortified—*not!* You love it. You make a getaway to the bathroom, he follows and has his way with you in the restroom stall. You resist, but he's too strong, and you don't resort to verbal protests because you don't want to cause a scene in public. You give in and allow yourself to be sexually dominated. (Bummer? Bet not!)

And, as promised, the taxicab sketch, dedicated to the debs: One of my rich preppy girlfriends shared a TMI tale about a racy incident of sober, S&M-y sex in a cab with her boyfriend. She told me they were in the middle of a lovers' fight and that he forced make-up sex right then and there as the taxi sped down the bustling New York City streets. She described it as "crazy, scary, and a lot of fun" and offered some tips. If you are considering this, I'd first size up the driver, and you must make sure the cab has a plastic divider between driver and naughty passengers (as all medallion cabs licensed by New York City do). I asked if the driver saw. She gave me a nervous laugh/shrug. "Well, he probably saw something but was too embarrassed to stare into the rearview. Alexis, it's not like you'll ever see the guy again, not like he'd like *care*, anyway, and in the city, tailgating drivers have enough to do jockeying for position and dodging the jaywalkers. Whatev." I suspect, for this cab driver, the action was tame compared to his prize Tales of the City. Prob rolled his eyes, just another day chauffeuring around the big city wacks. Certainly, if you go for it, you could dress up the scene with some whispered verbal role play and daintily coy sexual moves suited to the clandestine nature of the hookup. Consider: urban streets, after dark, taboo thrills "on the go"—Madame la Directrice just scored a film noir set, for free! No permit necessary.

Enhancements

This is the deal. I could give you a laundry list a gazillion examples long on how to decorate for every scene, just as I could hypothesize about possible scene locales and role-play moves, but that's not going to help you get from here to there. Your DSRP experience is going to feel forced and stagy unless the creative coordinates—the imagery, the scene-driving ideas, and the design work—are organically flaming from your own fantasy fire, not mine. That's why I've offered stories, not prescriptions, expecting that tales from the field will trigger and fuel your imagination. This isn't math class, where it's imperative that you adopt a set of firm, cold equations to "get it right." This is art class and today is Paint What You Want Day. The goal here is for you to read some juice and fill up enough that you can run with your own desires and creativity. Everyone dreams, fantasizes, and imagines, though in adulthood, the output sometimes gets repressed. So, rather than throwing down prescriptives, I offer instead some ideas you might find inspiring and helpful in moving you into the free-flowing state of openness and vulnerability that will intensify your movie.

Let's paint. Buy a shade of lipstick that's unusual for your makeup palette. Try killer red, or a soft nude color. Make Up For Ever (a chichi brand) just came out with a black lipstick. Wicked! Same goes for the eye shadows: Sort through the colors and don't be timid. Pick a look that you could *never* see yourself pulling off but have always wished that you could. (You can). Next time you're planning a night on the town, mentally flash on a snapshot of a celebrity or mannequin (a sexy punk chick, a Hollywood grande dame, a fantastical look on a runway model) and take that as inspiration for your face painting. Style your hair to fit the look, choose outfits from your closet, or buy something *so not you* to fit the fantasy image in your head. When you're all dressed and made up, snap a photo of yourself on your cell. Do a pose. Maybe choose the perfect backdrop in your own place. Maybe set design around its limitations. Make a character face: glam? rocker sneering cool? Monroe kiss pucker? a cold femme fatale? An elegant Princess Grace? Text the photo to your lover. Hell, post it on Facebook, Twitter, Instagram. Caption? Dunno . . . "My alter ego look"?

You're on a mission, but stressing over details will make it a chore. Take a night for yourself. Turn off the computer and the cell phone, tuck the kiddies and your kitty cat into bed, and take a long Monroe bath. A hot shower will work too. Get luxurious with it. Candles, wine (?), break out that French milled soap you got as a holiday present and tucked away for nights like tonight. Soak in the heat, release. Then like the sex goddess herself, slip into bed naked. Sleep completely in the nude. When asked what she wore to bed, Ms. Monroe once answered, "Why, Chanel No. 5, of course!" Movie star fluff aside, sleeping in the nude is more than just "natural-organic." It summons a sensual mix of feelings; you'll feel defenseless yet empowered by the sensation of wearing just you! It immediately engenders a sex goddess confidence and delicious freedom, like swimming in the nude. Oddly, given the vulnerability, when I sleep in the nude I tend to stretch out rather than tighten into the defensive fetal position. It sends me off to a lazy-sexy, gentle, and carefree place, and when I wake up, I feel like a naked forest nymph awakening from a sweetly rapturous slumber without a care in the world. As if placed on earth simply to be a goddess.

Music, Scents, and Mood Lighting

Music, low lighting, and seductive scents can turn even the most mundane rooms into fantasy palaces.

MUSIC

With music, the trick is to fit the rhythm to the tempo of the scene. Classical music might ruin your strip club/lap dance scene. Eighties dance club hits are all wrong for posh-woman-meets-the-cat-burglar. Sounds obvious, but your first impulse may be to select the tunes you dig rather than the ones that will drive the scene. If you're having trouble pairing music with your scene selection, remove yourself from the scene and assume the director's perch. Consider the situation objectively and creatively, imagining actors in the wings, awaiting your cue to immerse themselves in the scene. Now, as director, ask yourself which music speaks to you as the mood-maker. Are the actions of the characters bold and aggressive? Then pick hardcore rhythms. Is your scene languidly played, classically romantic? Then pick soft and nonintrusive sounds. The music can heighten the mood you want or it can fight with it. Don't be hasty, dialing up just any ol' radio station, because music also can be a great aid in calming nerves and "stage fright" jitters and in filling the awkward silence gaps that can break the spell during vocal role play. If you and your partner are better with actions than words, then crank up the record player. If it's your first time with a role-play scene and one or both of you is nervous or red-faced, crank it up with imposing sounds and let the music do the commanding.

LIGHTING

Pretty much across the play board, I recommend low lighting, and in this, candles are the bomb. Fire is a primal stimulus, guaranteed to elicit an emotional response. It can help diffuse stiffness and draw out dormant sexual impulses. Fire also creates an instant portal to fantasy land, flaming out the background noise and clutter of our humdrum existence. With the lights off, a candle used in an interrogation scene, or as illumination in a hostage scene—heavy bondage, you tied to a chair, perhaps—becomes an ominous spotlight on you, the captive, and can be your speedy ticket to that scary place. (Nothing scarier than a flash fire, however, and such scenes can be all-consuming, so beware!) Another lighting choice might be a construction site lamp, which you can buy inexpensively at hardware stores. Clip it onto a hanging light fixture, a curtain, a side table, or a lamp shade, and then just rearrange the furniture to make it work. Another transforming trick is to fit your fixtures with soft amber or blue-colored light bulbs. Red, as in red-light district, is good for a salty whorehouse scene, as any indie filmmaker could tell you. Break out the fishnets (tattered, of course) and the cheap stilettos and *wheeee!*

SCENTS

Smell is our oldest sense, and the right fragrance can evoke powerful and vivid memories. Scents work on the brain in mysterious ways, and, for this reason, you'll want to tread lightly and carefully—it won't do to conjure disagreeable reactions or (worse!) to summon the ghost of a long-lost love! You might invest in a sampler set of perfumes to start off your perfume wardrobe: something sexually provocative for Call Girl (Marc Jacobs's Oh, Lola!), classy for Classy Dame (Chanel No. 5, *bien sûr;*) madly wanton for The Vamp (is there a man on earth who doesn't respond to CK's Obsession?), sweet for The Virgin (Innocent by Thierry Mugler, gotta be, no?), and for Worldly Sophisticate, try Robert Piguet's Fracas, an intoxicating Parisian scent from the forties and one of my all-time faves. As with incense, which is used in meditation to slow the heart rate and calm aggressive impulses, most any sweet scent will help dispel anxiety and impulses that threaten to send the action into overdrive.

Romantic music, low lighting, and scented candles (or a drop of perfume applied to a *cold* bulb before lighting) can be used together as calming sensory aids—a one-two-three punch to take the edge off, soften the ambience, and slow the pace.

For fast-paced action scenes, let 'er rip! Amp up the heavy-beat music and bring out the firepower. We want him to *wake up* and behave as your sexual aggro beast. *Arrrrr!* Yum.

Take It from Mr. H: In Scene Play, No Drugs or Alcohol Allowed on the Set—Mean It!

One of the biggest temptations in DSRP (especially and understandably for beginners) is to knock back a drink or two before play. Booze is society's great loosening lager and, in this arena, seemingly a great way to break the ice. With your inhibitions down, your creativity will be freed and the good times will just roll, or so you might imagine. This, however, is sadly not the case. As with driving under the influence, you're at severe risk of running into walls, and that could ruin this kind of play for you for a long, long time. I've had some memorably bad experiences, in which everything seemed like a good idea at the time, and while I've had no disasters, the end results were less than pleasurable. Even worse, I've listened as others recounted nightmare scenarios in which drunken couples attempted things they shouldn't have, and wouldn't have, if booze or recreational drugs hadn't rearranged the perception and judgment centers of their brains. The atmosphere in a DSRP scene is, by nature and design, physically and emotionally intense. Restrictions apply and must be enforced. Consider the following four reasons to keep drugs and alcohol out of your role-playing adventures:

1. The most important thing at risk with the use of alcohol and drugs is the safety of the parties. Bondage, restraints, spanking, gags, and anything/everything else require that attention be paid during and, with certain items, in between sessions. DSRP hardware toys require inspection after each use and preventive maintenance to keep them in safe working condition. The last thing you need is to be judgmentally impaired while using restraints, as neither party will be able to gauge the proper fit; too tight, and the result can be bruising, cuts, or worse. No woman should be gagged or hooded and left alone. No drunk woman should *ever* be gagged, and under no circumstances should she consent to DSRP with a man impaired by drink or drug. I've heard of women being tied up and gagged, then left squirming by a passed-out play partner. In any case, bondage can be risky business and I would recommend to all safe practices (e.g., slipknots, keyed-alike padlocks, if chains are being used) and investment in equipment with uncoupling triggers, for use in case of emergency. My advice to men is to save the alcohol for the bar and the house party, and hit the bedroom with nothing but a traditional swagger, as these scenes require more work than you'll be able to put in if you're impaired.

2. Get even a bit tipsy, and the pacing of your scene will suffer, and nobody will be happy. Bottom line: Among new DSRP players, there is bound to be a certain amount of stumbling, awkward conversation, and outbursts of exasperation, even anger. All that is compounded when you're sloppily trying to negotiate each other's limits and figuring things out on the fly. Trust me, two of my worst scene experiences fell apart because my play partner and I were both inebriated. I won't give you a play-by-play, because it wouldn't even make a decent grade-C drunken frat boy comedy, but I can say this: Instead of sexual tension, we got arguments

and exhaustion, and everyone was pretty much completely unhappy by the end of the fumbling and bungling. Our scene idea sounded great in theory but quickly devolved into parody—two people trying to think way outside the box but landing on our asses inside the box, unable to save face or save the day.

3. What you say matters, and when you are impaired, verbal role play can get ugly quickly. Way happy or otherwise, nobody is a "good" drunk, and when put into an interplay where humiliation and insults commonly are used as "tweak" to the scene, one can easily go too far. Feelings will be hurt, explanations will be needed and demanded, and bad vibes are promised for the next morning. Not worth the trouble. Trust me.

4. Under the influence, both players risk doing things that are out of bounds: The dominant may overstep the sub's limits, and the sub may allow it. Both are sure to regret it. With your comfort levels compromised and your inhibitions down, can you be sure how you'll feel tomorrow about what you're doing tonight, and how taking liberties may reflect on you later? What might be exciting to you drunk may have long-lasting consequences when you've sobered up.

MY LAST WORD ON THE SUBJECT: Drinking and playing, like drinking and driving (and even drinking and dialing), has unforeseen consequences, none good. Beware.

Exercises

1. Yep. We are revisiting the source again: your erotic story or your chosen DRSP scene from a book or movie. Now we concentrate on the characters and scenarios, imagined or actual film scenes and sets. Pretend you've been hired to direct your fantasy role-play scene as a movie. Google image-search the character types or even the real film characters, and enter into your director's planning book details on costuming. Go to YouTube and watch the trailers from the movies that inspired your scene. Borrow from the masters.

2. Set design 101. Back to the computer. Google image-search your play scene set. These are terms I input and found fruitful: *brothel room*, *military encampment*, Secretary *film set Gyllenhaal, harem, seedy motel, Scarlett's bedroom*, and, not for the timid, *torture chamber* and *vampire castle* (can't you see Bram Stoker's Dracula as the perfect dom?). As you study the images, devise ways you can improvise. Red silk scarves draped over the bedroom lamps for the harem. Perfume bottles set up on the bureau and sex toys on the nightstands for the call girl's bedroom. Your computer desk outfitted with a fountain pen holder and a china cup and saucer for the big boss/secretary scene. (Hint: During play, make sure to get his coffee request all wrong so he has reason to bend you over the desk and . . . well, do you want a spanking punishment or a sexual tease?)

3. Visit the perfume counter of your favorite department store and pick out a character-appropriate fragrance, one that you've never used before. Ask for a sample and wear it during the scene. The idea here is to fool your senses into believing you're in that other reality. It will get you into character and damn well will get his attention. It's all in the pheromone scent research literature, and it's bloody primal, baby!

4. Download time. Like scent, ambient sound provides instant transport from reality to fantasy land. It also helps to cover up any nerves or "silencio." YouTube some songs you think will fit the mood of the scene. Listen to film soundtracks, find frisson-inducing songs, sample music outside your usual repertoire, from chanting Tibetan monks to punk rock. Now you can either play your song list during play or listen to select mood songs beforehand to prep yourselves, as actors do before diving into a scene.

AND WITH THAT, WE LEAVE THE realm of the senses and head into the fecund nothingness of sensory deprivation DSRP.

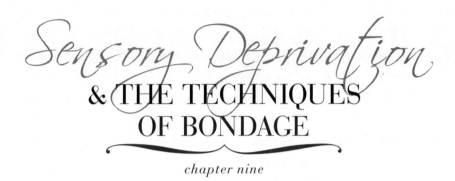

Sensory Deprivation
& THE TECHNIQUES
OF BONDAGE

chapter nine

Lord Ascot: Charles, you have lost your senses? This picture is impossible.
Charles Kingsleigh: Precisely. Gentlemen, the only way to achieve
the impossible is to believe it's possible.
—TIM BURTON'S *ALICE IN WONDERLAND* (2010)

What better motto to introduce the absolute upside-downness of a lose-your-senses concept like "deprive to enrich" than the whimsy of *Alice in Wonderland,* as imagined by the quirky director, writer, and visual artist Tim Burton?[1]

In sensory deprivation in the context of DSRP, one or more of a submissive's senses literally is deprived of input from the outside world. Her dominant deliberately cuts off (or dilutes) external stimuli in order to heighten her receptivity to touch and to intensify her sexual experience through the appetite-whetting ingredients of fear and anticipation. Articles of clothing such as blindfolds or hoods and earmuffs can be used to cut off sight and hearing. More complex devices can cut off the sense of smell, even touch, but in DSRP, why would your man want to do that?

In this chapter we will introduce sensory deprivation techniques and appropriate accouterments. You might read the chapter as a basic training manual for DSRP SD boot camp. From this material, a dominant may draw up a shopping list for his toolkit of devices and choose from the playbook of maneuvers, creating a combination that can cause . . . *fireworks!* Or, on the flipside, a Zen-like tranquility.

This yin and yang of sensory deprivation is a fascinating twofer. When you are in a physically vulnerable state, your yang-y dominant can easily provoke in you a thrilling fear of the unknown: Where is he, what's he plotting, what's he going to do, and *when will he "strike"?* If you're more in the mood for some yin-y mind games, he can play a gentler game of cat-and-mouse, feather-stroking and lulling you into a relaxed, meditative state.

The way you and your lover choose to use the devices/toys and play routines described in this chapter may depend on the mood of the day. Do you want sexual adrenaline pumps of roller-coaster extravaganza? Or is tonight the night for a relaxed slide into a Zen state of placidity, in which you float without worry, your alpha brainwaves converting to theta, a shift that normally occurs right before sleep and again before waking?

Note: Sensory deprivation, at *your* invitation and by *your* design, and explored in the company of a trusted partner, can be, at once, a stirringly scary proposition and an exhilarating adventure. But if practiced for extended periods of time, there can be negative psychological effects, so it's important to have your partner "watch the clock" and monitor your emotional state.

Let's look at two ways to play with sensory deprivation. Think back to your last trip to a carnival or amusement park. Did you beeline straight for the yang-y haunted house, eager for shocks and frights, with actors dressed up in horror costumes and masks, springing out unexpectedly to surprise, scare, and thrill you? Or did you stand in line for a yin-y gondola ride through the Tunnel of Love? A relaxing and romantic trip through the calm waters of a dark tunnel? Were you clenching his arm in the throes of fear as the masked monster-actors leaped out to surprise you? Or were you contentedly cooing with your lover in the womblike security of a darkened corridor? Or maybe you enjoyed both dark-passage carnival attractions? Of course you did! Both rides capitalize on the sensory deprivation technique of plunging you into darkness to heighten your receptivity either to scares or romance.

I've experienced and enjoyed both the cringing terrors and the soothing relaxation and file this report from the field. Let's take a walk to the haunted house of kink.

The Carnal Carnival

The art of kink role play can be a Picasso or a Monet. I prefer Picasso.

In describing *Picasso Érotique*, a 2001 exhibit at the Jeu de Paume Gallery in Paris, a reviewer for the *New York Times* observed, "By isolating his erotic works, this show is separating the inseparable: for Picasso, sex was as natural as painting. 'Art is not chaste,' he once said. 'It should be kept away from ignorant innocents. Those ill prepared should be allowed no contact with art. Yes, art is dangerous. And if it is chaste, it is not art.'" [2] *C'est exactement ça!*

There was nothing of the "vanilla world" about Picasso, not in his art, not in his life. Sex was ever-present in his works but, according to Dominique Dupuis-Labbé, a curator at the Musée Picasso, it became an overriding theme after his meeting with the seventeen-year-old Marie-Thérèse Walter (he was forty-five and married at the time), who became his muse and mistress. Dupuis-Labbé, the *New York Times* reviewer wrote, "said that [Picasso's] meeting with Walter in 1927 opened his second great period of erotic art. The bull, the centaur and finally the minotaur all made their appearance, variously representing the artist as both dominating and dominated. 'He was perhaps liberated from a certain frigidity,' Ms. Dupuis-Labbé said."

And thus may the sub liberate herself, becoming the artist "painting the scene" for her dominant. Both dominating (she's calling the shots) and dominated (by the bull/centaur/Minotaur figure of her creation), she immerses herself in the composition for a masked romp with her partner in their fantasy haunted house.

My Picasso-esque Scene

I had a long-enjoyed fantasy wherein my lover was an omnipotent being and I a powerless creature. Dressing the dude up in a police costume was not going to do it for me—too Chippendales or some eighties male stripper hoax comedy scene. Just couldn't get into the idea of costumes for him. (That's my kink hang-up, I hope not yours.) Most of my play scenes with Mr. H are designed by me and shipped off via email. I still prefer to hide behind my computer when *discussing* sex. Just call me a scaredy kink kitty. Meow-blush. I emailed him this proposed scenario:

> *Hey, I'm going to paint a hugely embarrassing scene, and if you are into it, all you gotta do is e-reply "Yes" with a time/date. Then you are to start organizing the scene and do as I have mapped out below. Sorry, no compromises on this one. If you're not into it, email me back: "Afraid." Because I will conclude that you are afraid, and that it is the thought of me, living through the terrors of the scene, that has you disturbed. If so, it's your problem, and I promise it will not be mine—IF you follow my instructions.*

> *The Scene: Interrogation*
>
> *You notice that I have left my Facebook page open to a conversation with a guy I had sex with one night after you and I fought. You confront me about the cheating and I deny it. (This isn't the time to come up with my disclaimers. I'll figure things out on D-day because I want it to sound—and be— spontaneous.) You then admit that you've seen my FB emails. You instruct me to undress to my lingerie (you can email me what type you prefer me to wear). Then you instruct me to sit down. You tie my ankles to the chair legs and bind my arms together in front of me—not behind me and not too tight. You may blindfold me with anything you want. I want you to interrogate me, drill*

*me about all the dirty details of each cheating incident. Be firm and threaten-
ing but nothing physically extreme. I want to feel that I have no control and to
feel genuinely scared of what you might do in your jealous "rage."*

Mr. H replied "Yes." And off we went.

ON THE DAY OF THE INTERROGATION, blindfolded with my own shirt and
tied to his dining-room chair, I listened as he stalked around me barefoot and came at me from different angles in erratic timeframes. I truly
felt a prisoner in a haunted carnival house and had not a clue when or
from which direction he was going to spring. Nor, good God, did I know
what he was going to do. I couldn't discern his movements, was literally
in the dark as to when he was going to pop up.

> *Mr. H: Did you suck his d***?*
> *Moi: You're a crude pig, how dare you . . . !*

Silence. Where was he? Had he left the room? Was he behind me,
ready to grab me by the hair? I was afraid, even though I knew myself
to be safe. Was he going to sexually assault me? Or had he decided
to abandon me here? I wouldn't call it passion exactly, or even excitement, but how to articulate what I was feeling? Hmmm . . . like a hot
tease? asking for rough sex? having flashes of second thoughts just before
impact? But! At the same time knowing it was going to be thrilling.

Tied to Mr. H's chair, I thought back to a field trip my class took to
a theme park (I must have been ten or so). A group of us (Ashley, Lind-
say, Yasmin, Jessica, and I) wandered off to the high cliff plunge fear
attraction. There was this surfer-blonde cool dude manning the death
dive, not at all pushy like some old-school carny barker, just chill and
friendly. The coast was clear to take the plunge—no line for *this* ride!
A group of people clustered six feet away from the cliff of thrills, each
flashing the same conflicting thoughts: *Should I or shouldn't I? Do I dare?*

All of my rogue prep gang decided no. I felt my palms sweat, my knees buckle, and even though I could see that I'd land safely in the pool of warm water, I thought, *No way!* The surfer dude said, "You could just jump from here," pointing to a lower cliff, but he didn't "push" anyone. I trusted him. I trusted *him*, as an individual, even though, being educated at an all-girls school, I hadn't yet gotten to know that creature called man. Still, I imagined that he'd have some power over me if I gave in to his suggestion and jumped. I knew if it had been a woman urging me to jump, scared or not, I would have done it. Jessica, my best friend at the time, braved up and said to the rest of us, "I know if I don't do it you'll all make fun of me." So off she went, eyes shut, like a blindfolded straight arrow, off the high cliff and into the abyss. We all scrambled down to the pool and waited for her to emerge. When she surfaced, she said, "It was great. But I would never do it again."(Jessica now lives in India where she runs her own charity, supplying village women with video cameras to record and share with the world their daily struggles and challenges.)

What made me, midscene with Mr. H, recall this childhood episode? I don't know, but I suspect that I was rethinking Jessie's own justification. I decided that, for her, it was less about the fear of being called a chicken and more about having the will to buck up and *be brave*, to dive in for the promised thrill of surprise. Similarly, my interrogation fantasy stemmed not from sexual desire but a readiness to experience the terror of the unknown, within the safe pool of play.

The Art of Creating Terror

Why does the DSRP player desire that her dominant perfect the adjunct art of creating suspense, fear, and surprise? According to Nan Wise, a sex therapist and neuroscientist who studies the brain at orgasm:

> *It's unpredicted stimuli that really fires up those dopamine receptors and gives you all that pleasure. So by exploring new things, including role play*

and BDSM, couples can re-engage the brain's reward centers, which may be habituated to doing the same kind of sex play over and over again.[3]

On this subject, I figure you'd like to see what a blogging dom is telling our men, so here I hand over the reins to Mr. H, who discusses the art of creating intimidation scenes employing sensory deprivation toys.

Mr. H: One of the most powerful illusions that can bring excitement and thrills to a scene is the creation of artificial danger. Sexuality and danger have always been connected, and if you can safely replicate the conditions that inspire fear/awe, you can also inspire greater sexual excitement and mystery in your scene. This part of the scene requires the most developed talents in terms of acting and delivery, but much like staging any movie or play, the power will build as you develop your skills and begin to add your own little touches that make the action *seem* real because it *feels* real. Here are a few techniques I've picked up along the way to hone your craft in creating a sense of playful aggression and fear in your personal play. Once your partner is bound, she is at your mercy, but to make her *believe* she's at your mercy and not just "tied up by Mr. Same-o Same-o Tried and True," use any of the following suggested techniques to heighten her fear and awe of you, to build respect for your fearsome power, and to bend her to your will.

While she is blindfolded, with or without sound deprivation (earplugs or an iPod for the submissive):

HAIR PULLING

Hair pulling is often seen as a "heat of romance" thing, but when you are bound, gagged, and blindfolded, it is a physically dominating experience that invades your whole being, causes (in tolerable amounts) pain, and wrecks the hairdo—to most women, a sacrosanct trademark of their presentation. Being incapacitated, when she feels the hair pulling and hears your whispered "not to worry" transmitted directly into her ear, trust me, she's going to start worrying! In grabbing a chunk of her hair, you'll also control the movement of her head. It's a rough and intimidating action but causes no real harm (just keep things under control, folks) and can be a great addition to the fear-building aspects of the verbal play.

FACE SLAPPING

This is one spicy-hot method of intimidation. As Alexis has written, from the sub's POV, it needn't (and shouldn't!!!) be done harshly to qualify as a great attention-getter that will keep the submissive off-balance. A good smack in the face can turn a defiant partner into a partner who continues to behave, simply because, to her mind, that smack in the face is always just around the corner. I can think of many strong, defiant types who calmed down after a few smacks to the face and complied nicely and left with no physical harm done. It's not the smack, per se, but rather the unexpected invasion of the sub's "personhood," with a gesture that stings (the self and the pride) and stuns just enough to remind her who's in control here. If you can't see when one of these smacks to the face is coming (in cases of blindfold play), can't avoid the smacks (due to bondage), and can't talk back to beg a halt (due to a gag), these slaps create a great sense of discomfort, worry, and fear that can be exploited on a regular basis.

KNIFE/GUN PLAY

The use of weapons (fake in the gun department—try a prop shop) can heighten the tensions in a bound experience. When you can't move, speak, or ignore the presence of a knife gently touching the skin or a gun (once again, replicas **only**) put to the back of the head, weapons play makes one helluva real impression, believe me. The pressure of a cold, sharp object against the skin, or the fearsome presence of a gun, can send the imagination into overdrive, creating worry and fear in a way other tools won't. If used menacingly but cautiously (in the case of a sharp blade), weapon wielding can be a great addition to any script with villain play. In a scene with a street thug holding up his captive or a robber trying to force his victim to tell him where the valuables are hidden, these intimidating tools can help deliver the goods. As in all exploits, practice makes perfect, so be sure both of you know what you're doing before you introduce this kind of play into your work; no sudden moves from either side of a sharp blade. The play prop pistol can be pressed up against a body part so that the submissive is made to feel the barrel. Feeling can elicit more blood-pumping terror than seeing in a blindfolded submissive.

VERBAL PLAY

The power of the human voice is, of course, your most easily accessed and useful accessory weapon. Whispering threats and insults is a great way to intimidate and fluster a bound captive. If she is gagged, this is a one-way conversation, if you don't count a muffled "mmmmph." With this as her only possible verbal response, the dom is free to further taunt and bully, mocking even her pathetically feeble protest. Inflicting believable threats, and using your practiced I-will-be-obeyed delivery and tone of voice, will serve as powerful backup to any of the other techniques designed to break the will. Be harsh and evasive, come at her from different angles so that she's always left to wonder where you're standing. In negating various senses, you create a mood in which every threat, every insult, and every act of intimidation becomes convincing reality. It's one thing to say, "I'm going to slap you if you don't stop moving," to someone free to move, but when bound, all they can do is "watch" and wait in fearful anticipation. And with the imposing voice, the foreboding becomes unbearable.

BLACKMAIL/FEAR OF EMBARRASSMENT

That whole "if you don't respect my authority, you're gonna get it" thing, and, yeah, any of the above techniques, don't come close to inspiring the fear of a public humiliation. Taking pictures of the submissive on a cell phone and letting her know that you might just post it online or send it to a mutual friend can be the compelling proper motivator. Also fun is to keep said images and encourage "repeat" performances of the scene, under the pretense that you might post these images, unless she continues to submit to your wishes and desires. Think ruthlessly: "Remember that photograph I have of you, hog-tied and with myself in your mouth? Let's make an appointment . . ." Of course this is all role play (or *should* be), and it's you and your partner's job to allow that fantasy to seem a reality. Her fear of the world's seeing her tied up, compounded by her recalling an even fiercer struggle when the camera came out, will serve as a real fear-creating experience. Only a despicable cad would break the bonds of friendship and loyalty in releasing such images, but, still, the web is full of evidence that cads abound. Obviously, trust is all important here.

[A "cover your ass" note from Alexis: Mr. H talks up the idea of picture-taking and dangling as a means of creating positive tension, but personally I find this a first-class lousy idea *unless it's done on your own equipment*. That way, you can let him shoot and threaten away during your play scene, and when the curtain falls, you may sweetly ask to reclaim your cell phone. Mr. H is a good guy, not a cad, but as he says, cads abound . . . 'sides, I have known him to misplace his iPhone.]

Just remember though, the idea in sensory deprivation play, as in all DSRP, is to create fear through innuendo and illusion. The experience may be likened to that of a ride on a world-class roller coaster: The thrill is in the terrifying demonstration of "risk" though the "risk" doesn't actually exist—not, that is, for the prudent thrill-seeker who respects the dangers and plays by the rules, strapping in and safely enjoying the hell out of a bloodcurdling ride. Similarly, being tied up isn't a dangerous proposition if you trust your "tormentor." By applying some tried-and-true, angst-provoking techniques, however, you can twist and turn a romantic bondage encounter into a blockbuster his-and-hers night to remember.

A Monet Sensory Deprivation Scene

My first experience with DSRP sensory deprivation, well before I had any real knowledge of BDSM, or even that there was a BDSM scene, was when I was a ferocious student of yoga. I got a monthly membership to a new yoga school on the Upper East Side of Manhattan and took two classes a day. That was three hours of sweaty, bendy yoga every day. Sitting cross-legged, all perked up and nervous about my first encounter with a male yoga instructor, I was disarmed when he skipped into the room. He turned out to be a slight-framed yogi in his midthirties, with big-rimmed glasses and a goofy gait. His easy self-confidence and humility couldn't hide the unmistakable aura of high intelligence. All of these qualities worked to soften my unease at the prospect of being touched and physically molded into yoga pose adjustments by a *man*. I have always been yoga teacher Play-Doh, as I'm abnormally physically flexible. On this occasion, the teacher's hands were firm, confident, and unforgiving as he pushed down on my ass to force the spread of my legs from a half split to a full-to-the-ground split. He wasn't aggressive but insistent that "yes, you can" push farther and grind down into the floor. That's when the pings of pain sparked up and just as quickly died out, like embers, leaving a lukewarm pleasure-pain sensation that swirled around my pelvis region. It hurt so good, and not in a masochistic way (I have somewhat less than zero pain tolerance, BTW). The first jolts of pain boiled over into truly orgasmic ping sensations in my groin. Wow!

(Note to the reader: These yogis court pain way beyond that solicited by BDSM subs. I've seen more yoga practitioners, at the mercy of said yogis, hurt themselves and sustain permanent, doctor's-office-visit-worthy injuries than I ever saw among subs in my dominatrix dungeon days. Yogis and kinksters, hmmm . . . However, unlike BDSM practitioners, yogis who punish themselves and end up suffering self-inflicted knee injuries and ripped ligaments, often defying doctors' orders to stop, are not persecuted by the press. And in instances when a groaning pupil suffers injury as a result of being encouraged by a teacher to "push further," neither is the yogi subject to punishment under the law. Waving fingers, I know, but it grates.)

Back to what I now consider my first experience with sensory deprivation. After the bending, sweating, and stretching, the yoga students lie down for *Savasana*. This is the Corpse Pose, the ritual ending to every yoga class, in which everyone lies on the back, legs apart, palms facing up, and eyes closed. Full submission to the cosmos. *Oooo la la*. Like a good yogini chick, I try to do as bidden: keep my eyes closed, lie on my back, completely still, not let my thoughts wander to the pressing question of whether the yoga teacher has decided he wishes to try to have his way with me.

Yes! He does. He creeps softy to my mat, barefoot, "on little cat feet," and starts to pinch my ears softly. I continue to observe end-of-yoga-class rituals. The ears, I learn from Mr. H seven years later, are an erogenous zone (erectile tissue, actually). I was feeling it. Then the instructor (this is just after he's gently pushed my body into extreme pelvis-opening stretches) whispers in my ear, "You have a beautiful practice." I'm strung out from the painful stretching; I'm feeling the effects of the endorphins released by the pain; physically, I'm in a vulnerable, blinded position; and I'm sexually stimulated from the ear caressing/pinching. I choke up in near tears of I don't know what, but it's lovely.

"Are you all right?" I manage a faint "Yes." He presses a single finger between my breasts. I'm blinded and confused, but it's yoga class . . . but he's a *man* . . . *eeeek?* He retracts the finger, and I'm not sure if he's gone away or if he's still hovering. I feel what I take to be a ghost presence of his finger above my chest . . . am I imagining? I'm not. His finger firmly but slowly presses down between my breasts again. He continues to whisper sweet, calming words into my ears, while gently pinching them and sending my body into an unmistakable state of sexual arousal.

He never crossed any yoga instructor line of ethics in class, but we did plunge into a tantric sex affair, starting, well, after that class. It lasted months and ended when I found out that he had lied to me, was, in fact, married with a child. Mr. H, a professed male dominant, does not lie to women and is never anything but up-front and straight up about his dominant desires and his relationship status. Yes, the small and gentle yogi lied, and the six-foot-four Viking dominant scaryman, admittedly and wholeheartedly into BDSM, misleads no one and never hurt me a smidge.

But that's not the point of my story about the instructor. The yogi dominant dommed me in an ethical, nonsexual way in that class, and yes, it was a form of DSRP. Mr. H has tied me up, blindfolded me down, and given me a scalp, ear, and back massage while whispering erotic tunes and sending me off into the exact same submissive state— allowing me to master me and feel at once relaxed and stimulated. No cliff-jumping jitters but a spiky sense of "what is the dominant going to do, be, say, next?" while I'm blind, helpless, and under his control. A peaceful yet vibrant Monet painting, the yin of sensory deprivation DSRP.

THE BONDAGE BODY MASSAGE

Here, Mr. H discusses the bondage body massage with the guys.
His invention. C'est magnifique!

Mr. H: While many people are curious about exploring restraint-based fantasies, the idea of simply meeting someone to explore these concepts (even on a nonsexual basis) is a bit intimidating. For someone who might have played with handcuffs with a former boyfriend (at best), the idea of acting out an entire scenario involving full bondage and role-playing with a new partner may give pause. Simply, she may see it as "too much too soon." As with anything that challenges boundaries, pushes limits, and requires surrendering some degree of control, she may feel the need first to become comfortable in her relationship with you before exploring your kinky interests.

In the past few years of studying and developing these ideas, I've found a user-friendly first step that has become one of the more popular suggestions. This allows one to dip a toe into the world of restraint without requiring the complex role play that often fails in a beginners' setting. (This often occurs even if one person is experienced and the other is not, as it can take a great deal of time to develop the trust, rhythm, and know-how needed to pull off a complicated and theatrical scene.) This concept, mixing massage and bondage, crosses into both camps, allowing for a delicate, pleasurable baby step into the realm.

This particular scenario offers a combination of sensations and visuals that can please both parties and dispel the nerves that beginners may feel about both practices. It should be thought of as a Bettie Page–type of scene in which you can mix elegant clothing, complex yet comfortable restraints, and a moderate level of tension. This will make for a scene that almost any two people can enjoy, no matter what their levels of experience in bondage and role-playing.

Here I will provide a breakdown of suggestions and background information on how to make this mixture of bondage and massage easy, fun, and a great first step for those wishing to indulge their curiosity.

THE BASICS

This kind of scenario is as easy as they come. There is no opening scene, no closing scene, and the dialogue can be kept to an absolute minimum. The concept is very simple: the irresistible massage that *cannot* be resisted. The mood should always be playful, the bondage applied with little in the way of resistance, with comfort being the main goal.

THE COSTUMES

Here you can have a bit of extra fun. As this is not a character-specific scene, it allows the freedom to wear anything you want, but as it is sensual role play, the idea should be to present the female counterpart as being as beautiful as possible. One key aspect of the psychology of these kinds of bondage scenes is that, even subjugated, underneath all the rugged bondage materials, a woman wants to feel beautiful. After all, the practice of bondage in one's personal life is not about abuse but rather a resetting of the primal male-female dynamic. During DSRP sessions, the female partner is brought under the control of her male counterpart, taken charge of *and* taken care of, in whichever ways—sexual or sometimes not—the couple has chosen.

TONE SETTING

So, in this scene, think elegant and classy. Glamour can be a great tool in creating the proper tension between the sexes and especially here, where the woman is encouraged to get herself "all dressed up with no place to go." Even if the scene is to be a platonic encounter, she will feel more attractive and the visual attraction will be more enticing for the individual providing the massage. Also, the more she wears in the beginning, the better, as it will allow for a little playful struggle, and the longer it takes to remove her clothing, the more the drama builds. A good rule of thumb is to begin the massage with her fully clothed, concentrating first on the few exposed areas. Then you may begin the leisurely process of disrobing her, which will add to her feeling of vulnerability. Also, remember to rearrange the bondage every now and again so that she experiences no discomfort.

THE INTERPLAY

While a prepared script isn't needed, some amiable interplay can maximize the potential of a simple and enjoyable silent massage with ropes and one or more SD accessories. It will be a one-way conversation carried by the person providing the massage, engaging his restrained and silenced massage partner. It's best, in such a scene, to avoid being crass. Rather, one can initiate playful banter with some gentle ribbing and the paying of compliments. You can also build the scene by announcing your intentions before committing the action. If you're planning to remove an article of clothing, you can tease the action in advance. Even if you've played masseuse to this partner before, the fact that this time you and you alone are determining the routine and the pace can provide an edge to the interplay that gently pushes the boundary, creating anticipation and putting you firmly in control. It can also be interesting to make the person aware of her restrained position, gently prodding her verbally as you perform the rubdown.

Remember, this is a lighthearted scene, and since none of it relies on any kind of force, it's best to establish control using mild measures to convey your firm but giving domination in the situation.

THE TECHNIQUE

While most people know how to give a basic massage, in this it's as much about pacing and drama building as it is about giving a basic back rub. If you've never provided a full-body massage, it might be best to look up some of the finer points and get in some practice, to ensure that every part of the body receives a workout. This allows two people to become physically intimate in what for both of you may be a brand-new approach to foreplay.

THE BONDAGE

In a scene like this, the restraints should be both comfortable and just restricting enough to prevent escape without making it impossible for the two of you to switch positions. Silk or satin rope is the ideal restraint, as it's gentle yet holds its own against a good struggle. The good old "fuzzy" handcuffs can be employed to both ankles and wrists for maximum effect. (One should buy about five pairs, in various sizes, so that they may be employed in different positions).

In theory, the best bondage for this sort of scene is the simplest: the arms bound firmly behind the back and the legs together side by side. If done properly, this will provide just enough resistance to be exciting but will allow a full range of motions for the massage. If, along the way, you feel the need for a greater challenge, you can remove the bonds and try a few different positions, e.g., a chair tie or a hogtie, so that you can access the legs and have maximum access to the back.

If she is to be gagged, a simple, small ball gag will do the trick. (No kink stores in the neighborhood? No worries. Amazon has gotten with the program and offers a full range of kink toys.) If she is new to this and prefers a familiar substitute, a silk scarf (across the mouth or drawn between the lips, called a cleave gag) will work while allowing her suppressed communication. Remember, keep it simple, keep it comfortable.

THE "P-GAG"

Rarely discussed, rarely used for any dramatic effect, and one of the most interesting choices of restraint is the female undergarment. (Yes, folks, that's right—the panties. There, I said it. Even I had a hard time with that one . . .)

In discussions regarding the elements of a potential scene, few proposals evoke the same jolt, curiosity, resistance, and tentative interest than the use of someone's undergarments to restrain her verbally. Why is that so? Symbolically, the female undergarment in question represents the feminine wile. It's the seducer, it's the defender, it can create a reaction simply based on its looks, and, most meaningfully, it occupies the space between what the outside world gets to see and what the wearer herself doesn't even see. It's the first thing she puts on, the last thing she takes off. If panties didn't hold such subtle psychological power, lingerie designers wouldn't dream up countless hundreds of variations and women wouldn't own drawerfuls in all colors, shapes, and styles.

It's one thing to restrain someone, another to add elements of the restraint that push the unbalanced nature of the roles. Using someone's own underwear as a verbal restraint pushes the equation of "I need to silence you" to "I am going to silence you unnervingly." Applying this common symbol of female sensuality, privacy, and mystery to silence her makes the deeper emotional point to the bound party as to her place in the scene, her total capitulation. When the undergarment seen as the shield between your most vulnerable and "protected" spot (and still illegal to display in an establishment that serves alcohol) is turned into a tool of submission, it fires the triggers that spell exciting, dangerous, and edgy.

APPLICATION AND SAFETY

Using a pair of panties is no different from using any other form of gag in which cloth stuffing is used to increase the silencing effect. That being said, a pair of female undergarments is shaped differently from a small hand-cloth or scrap and can be more difficult to prepare for placement into the mouth. The selection of a proper pair should be based not only on attractiveness but also functionality. A full panty may be too cumbersome to allow the binding elements to be properly secured. A tryout is recommended. Also, avoid panties with ribbons, lacy flaps, or buttons, which could detach and become lodged in the throat.

Finit: Be safe, watch your knickers, and happy hunting .—Mr. H

Bondage Positions and Style Techniques

All right, the art of bondage started in Asia with a Japanese technique called *shibari* that requires years of intense training to master. There are tons of *shibari* books out there. If you want to spend a lo-o-o-o-ng time (way too long, to my mind) learning how to be tied up in visually artistic ways, go for it. I decided to not cover the *shibari* technique in any depth, as it's way too complex and tedious to learn and, in my experience, the tie-up takes so long to do that it ruins the momentum and visceral passion of the scene, particularly the tying action, which is exciting when done at an aggressive pace. I know this is an invitation for *shibari* practitioners and authors to shoot hexes at me, shriek curses, unearth mummies, write imprecations in blood, and stab skinny blond voodoo dolls with a hundred pins. Pffft! Though I will say, *shibari* feels great for full-body suspension. In that practice, the dominant spends an hour securely tying you up, *shibari*-style, on a suspension rig so that you can hang and feel like you're floating. I doubt that's going to happen in your living room. Unless you go hog wild at the kink store and buy a suspension rig (one that comes with a *shibari* master to kink you up!). If you want to experience that, easier to attend a kink party in your area and volunteer to be suspended. (A website dedicated to finding area kink parties, from underground to large commercial ones, is also provided in chapter 12.)

Short of becoming a *shibari* master, there are plenty of easier techniques to learn and execute. Here are a few of them.

Wrists, Knees, and Ankles

Legs tied to chair or bed posts. Arms to chair or bedposts. Or arms tied to legs. Having your knees tied is cool for spanking or for feeling completely captured and bound, but it's hard for your lover to get in between your legs. (Might be a problem?) Alternatively, you can have your arms or wrists tied with a long rope, which then is secured to the sturdy base of a chandelier or a chinning bar apparatus. With the rest of your body firmly grounded (or bedded), you can enjoy a halfway-hanging sensation.

Asymmetrical bondage (equilibrioception)

Wherein a person is tied in asymmetrical positions, e.g., one arm is tied to the leg on the same side, or one ankle is tied to the thigh of the same leg, confusing the body's sense of balance. The disorienting effect increases the psychological impact of the bondage. Google *asymmetrical bondage* and you'll find tons of odd and creative ways to play with this technique, which is common in the art of Japanese bondage. I'm not a fan, as it sparks up my claustrophobic issues, but don't count it out. Many subs have told me that it intensifies the effect of bondage, that it is a welcomed mind-fuck, as the body has trouble adjusting to anything asymmetrical. They say it heightens the feeling of vulnerability and submission and is good for people with overactive, racing brains who get easily bored or have trouble settling into the scene. Asymmetrical bondage creates a brain-off effect as it coaxes you into concentrating on your physical state rather than on your racing thoughts, which can interfere with your connection to the scene and your lover.

Collar bondage

I'm not into collars either, because they can feel a bit too overwhelming, physically and mentally, and I wouldn't recommend collaring for your first trip to the rodeo. If collars seem a turn-on to you, or if you've played with them before, try one on and wear it around the house for a few hours. (This, in fact, is a good tip for a first-time use of any toy. You don't want to be stuck in a scene, possibly frantic and regretting having yielded to your dom's taste in toys. As with an unfamiliar dish served at the dinner party, be polite, give it a taste . . . not for you? Give it a "no thanks.") If you're not a fan of the collar but your partner continues to plead for it (guys really seem to go for that "leashed" look), here's my advice: Suggest that he might find the playmate he seeks at a pet store. If he's a sport (Posh Girls like good sports), he'll give you a "hardy har har" and move on. Not put off by the collaring idea? Then you'll be delighted to find that there is a wide variety of kink collars available, ranging from cheapo functional to high-end glam, even custom models studded with diamonds (for the posh pet, perhaps? Ha.) Your dominant can wrap the collar around your arm or leg, even your waist if you're built like our girl Miz Scarlett.

Full Arm Restraints

These full hand and arm "gloves," usually made of leather, can be found at kink stores. They can be more comfortable than a wrist tie, as they don't inflict pressure on a single area.

Full Hand Mittens

Also found at kink stores, these are for bad sub kitties with a history of testing their dominants in escape attempts. Like the full arm glove, the mitten does the trick for both partners: They work, and they don't tax the wrists. There are tons more hardcore and bizarre kink store items, but many belong on the extreme shelves and may seem too kinky-weird to the player who's not into (or not far into) the whole BDSM closet of devices. I'll discuss some of the hardcore goods in chapter 12, which is all about taboos.

The Hogtie

Round her up, cowboy! Jeez, that name, *hogtie*, is too much, but don't let that ick you. This hardcore yet popular bondage position can be seriously erotic. Usually, with you lying on your stomach, your dominant ties your arms to your legs, behind you, creating a circle with your body. In yoga practice, it's called the Bow Pose (*Dhanurasana*), as in the archer's arsenal, and yes, sometimes yogis use straps to pull their arms and legs together further. In fact, the bondage version is a position you can relax into much more so than the yoga version, as you don't have to strain to hold your legs and arms together—the ropes do it for you.

FYI: The hogtie/bow pose position is said to offer the following health benefits:[4]

- Warms and strengthens the entire body, mostly the legs, back, and buttocks
- Massages the abdominal organs

- Aids digestion
- Is therapeutic for those with respiratory ailments
- Fights fatigue
- Counters anxiety
- Stretches and opens the whole anterior spine
- Improves posture

Okay, I'm hereby renaming the DSRP hogtie. Henceforth, it will be the "bow tie." Much more civil, no?

The erotic benefits of the bow tie are that it gives your dominant full access to your spicy body parts, and it limits your ability to struggle. Sometimes, I feel compelled to struggle when restrained in a less intensive bondage position, because I feel that if I'm able to struggle, I must! Not to look *too* damn submissive to my partner. Given my scrappy personality, imagining myself in an actual captive situation, I feel fury and fight like mad for my freedom, with predictable results: I screw up a perfectly delightful scene.

Alexis Talks Toys

You can't imagine what the kink designers are imagining these days! I mean, to-tweet-about *gorgeous*! (Prices to match, I would add). I saw a kitten-themed blindfold mask complete with gold-tipped ears in German *Vogue* this spring (March 2013), featured in an *editorial*, not an ad, and I'm telling you, the full force of the shot screamed not kink but HAUTE COUTURE. The stunning name-brand model was in an I-can't-*live*-without-that-little-black-dress number, styled to the heights of Fashion Heaven like a spread for the House of Balenciaga (or Valentino, or . . . fill in the blank). Breathtaking. And for anyone still wondering if Anastasia Steele has arrived, this million-dollar shot says *yes*, she has!

For those who shy away from kink store devices—too pricey, unsure the commitment is long-term—no worries. We have you covered. *Wink

Blindfolds

THE LINGERIE BLINDFOLD: You don't need to hit the kink store, as almost any undergarment can be tied to form a homemade blindfold. In fact, some people find it more erotic to use intimate clothing as a play device. I recommend it.

THE EYE MASK, HOME-STYLE: You can always slap on the ol' generic sleepy. If you favor a special purchase and a shopping trip, visit the kink store—and be prepared to be dazzled! (Note: Online kink stores are listed in the appendix.)

THE KINK-WORLD EYE MASK: Kink store eye masks tack on the coolest tidbits to the trusty sleep mask. Several models are trimmed with faux fur that feels delish on the eyes. Harsher leather masks (think the Hannibal Lecter getup) are designed to intensify the aura of intimidation in play.

THE FULL HOOD: You can find leather hoods ranging from models with full mouth and nose breathing slits to ones with just hole pokes for nose breathing. You can also opt for a combo hood and ball gag. I would not recommend any full-headed hoods for anyone remotely claustrophobic (like *moi*). But full hoods certainly enhance the sensory deprivation experience, as they intensify feelings of helplessness, isolation, and vulnerability and assuredly help you tune out and let go.

Gags

THE LINGERIE GAG: The panty gag I would rally for. It's the most taboo and most titillating (as Mr. H explained earlier in this chapter). Otherwise, you can use a bra, stockings, garter belt, etc.

THE MEN'S TIE GAG: *Fifty Shades*–style. This is great if you've chosen a dominant character who is urbane, debonair, and sophisticated, not a Tarzan type or the ill-mannered burglar.

THE BALL GAG: Kink stores have a wide range of ball gags, with small to large balls. Pick your size. But! Warning: Red Flag Alert! *Do not go cheap with ball gags*. Buy one made of silicone. The problem with cheaper models is that they are made of rubber (like a pencil eraser), which tastes awful, and the gag *literally* will make you gag. Ugh. Also, the attachment sides of a cheap ball gag are poorly designed and can be very rough and uncomfortable. They will hurt the sides of your mouth. The pricier ones are worth every dollar because they're made of higher-grade materials that are tasteless, and they have been carefully designed so that the sides are ultra smooth with no hard edges so that your mouth is protected. Look for ball gags with rounded, smooth-surfaced mouth side guards.

THE SOFT ROPE GAG: Kink stores sell a silky smooth rope with the feel of a drapery cord. Soft rope is a hot combo: In appearance, it does the trick as the secure bondage choice, while in performance, it softens the blow. The captive sub experiences the erotic feeling of being restrained but she suffers none of the pain of being rubbed raw by a hardware store industrial rope.

THE HARDWARE STORE ROPE GAG: Or maybe you *want* the rough, full, real-deal stuff to render the captive scene more believable and sexually intense for you? (There's a name for this: It's called rough rope play . . . *duh*.) The hardware store on the corner has just what you're looking for. Prickly, hurty.

THE DUCT TAPE GAG: What *can't* you do with this stuff? Our motto in college was, "If you can't duct it, fuck it!" I would suggest a *small* piece of duct tape. Work out the length beforehand so that the tape doesn't trap and pull out your hair. Ouch! Also: You can get a full-blown movie robbery scene feeling using duct tape, but make a slit in the tape so that you can breathe through your mouth.

Restraints

THE LINGERIE RESTRAINT: Hands and feet can be tied with stockings, bras, garter belts, even a G-string. But be aware that most lingerie ties are easy to get out of and a slip-out could ruin your bondage scene.

THE MEN'S TIE RESTRAINT: *Fifty Shading* it again. Great for a simple hands or feet tie. I would stay away from using more than one tie. The power of using a man's tie lies in the fact that it's *his* tie. He's wearing it, and he takes it off to tie you up, to get the job done. Otherwise the tie has no intrinsic sexy symbolism; it might as well be a scarf or a piece of nondescript cloth. If you don't want to go bondage shopping, yeah, haul out his tie rack and make your choice. Just make sure he's wearing it on the night of the grand event.

THE NONSTICK TAPE RESTRAINT: This totally cool product is made especially for the bondage crowd. It sticks to itself without hair/skin-pulling glue. Your dominant can even wrap this tape around your face (and hair) for an interesting improv gag or full-headed hood experience. It's very soft and sensual. If shopping online, search for *bondage tape*.

THE ROPE RESTRAINT: Again, if you want the full-on captive experience, any hardware store will have skeins of horror film-worthy rope. Very few people I know go that far, but the roughness of the rope sure does add a dose of reality to the captive scene fantasy. Don't try it if it's your first time playing. Nothing like a painful freakout to spoil a playnite. Better for the new initiate to use the soft, silky rope sold in kink stores (see above under gags).

HANDCUFFS: Yes, for this, you must head to the kink store. Do not get cop handcuffs from the Halloween store. They're for show, not meant for play, are uncomfortable, and can be hard to get out of (you might have to call the fire department for a rescue, though it wouldn't be the strangest challenge they've ever answered). Kink store handcuffs are designed with safety releases or come with keys. Being disorganized, I've spent maddening hours searching for the key ("#%$&! Where the hell? F*ck! 911!"). So be safe and get a pair that your dominant can release with the push of a button on the cuff. Or put the key in a place you and he choose; put Post-It notes around the apartment reminding you where the hell the key is; have your guy wear it around his neck like a dog collar. I like that.

THE PUFFY CUFF: There are comfortable handcuffs made of fabric. You may consider it a problem, however, that they won't have the look or feel of the real deal.

THE POSH CUFF: More and more high-end kink sites are popping up for our posh pleasure. *Bon Dieu*! Even Louis Vuitton is out with couture play cuffs (pssst, Madonna got her LVs in gold). Or you can find glamour cuffs made of real fur (I'm a posh PETA girl, so I'm not hot to promote this item). More couture-fare websites in the appendix.

Miscellaneous Sensory Deprivation and Enhancement Devices and Techniques

EAR PLUGS/EAR MUFFS: Used to drown out outside sound stimuli for a more relaxing experience in soft role play or a more thrilling and angsty adventure, as your inability to locate your partner through the sounds of his movements will add to your feelings of isolation and vulnerability.

IPODS/MUSIC: Music drowns out the peripheral sounds as effectively as earplugs. A soundtrack filling your consciousness can help submissives who have racing brains, with thoughts firing continuously, and who find it hard to tune in and connect with the scene action. Also a good approach if your dominant sucks at, or is nervous or embarrassed about, verbal role play. Knowing that you've tuned him out will relieve him of the responsibility to come through with the repartee.

THERMOCEPTION: This is one of our senses that generally we're reminded of only *in extremis*. It sorta just hums along on the back burner until we inadvertently land a pinkie finger on the back burner, and then *ouch!* You got it, that's our thermoception talking to us. Your dominant can make creative use of your thermoception with harmless temperature shocks—not ouchy but surprising.

ICE: An ice cube to the stomach (or nipples or V-spot), yow! And blindfolded, the submissive can't distinguish between freeze and burn shocks (you know how that goes), which translates to a wake-up summons and, shall we say, collects the thoughts and reminds that your lover/dom is calling the shots.

HEAT/FIRE PLAY: Okay, I'm not getting crazy. I'm not talking about burning, as in blisters and pain. Oh, noooo, we are using fire to warm, not to hurt. Your dominant may warm his hands under the hot-water faucet or over the kitchen burners and then touch them to the areas he just flash-froze. Some women like to have candle wax dripped onto their bodies, but suggest this *only* after first trying it on yourself! If this appeals, look into the slow-drip play candles available through the online kink store. Otherwise, have him raise the candle high above you (to allow the wax to cool a bit on its way to the target) and carefully control the pace of the drips. Hey, the kink stores have a huge color selection, which could turn your wax play into a Jackson Pollock body painting. How chichi cool is that? (BTW: I've seen photos of amazingly beautiful wax play art on subs, some resembling sixties pop-art works from Andy Warhol.)

As a way to control your urge to squirm or tussle, your dom can allow a candle flame to get *near* your body—but never touching! Eeeek! Don't use a torch or incense burner or lighter—too dangerous. This takes steady nerves and a cautionary warning on his part, but, even then, he must be careful as hell and both of you must observe the "absolutely no drinks before fire/heat play" rule. No two-drink maximum here; bar is *closed* for you.

FURRY FABRICS: Kink stores sell furry gloves, or you can use any furry or faux fur piece of clothing that feels great on the body. Especially after a nipple pinch or a spank on the arse, the pleasure-giving follow-up is good for balance. Soft after heavy. But more on that later.

FOOD PLAY: Having your dominant feed you while you're blind-folded can be a great move for the gentle, nurturing dominant character (daddy?) you've chosen. Pick decadent foods: fruit, chocolate, caviar, oysters, desserts, something extravagant and erotic. Even if he's a meat-and-potatoes kinda guy, remember, this is about *you*, and I can't see that meatloaf and low-sodium chickpeas are going to do it.

SMELL: For a more relaxed scene, enhance the slow-paced soft role play with some incense in scents known to be soothing: lavender or san-dalwood, for instance. This will calm you and your dominant. A great unwinder for tightly coiled players.

A Final Thought on Bondage and Sensory Deprivation

Through the confinement of bondage, with blindfolded eyes, you may log off your five-sense reality and shift your focus inward. Freed from the distractions of external visual stimuli, in fact you have nowhere else to "set your sights," and, paradoxically, this can be an eye-opener. You actually begin to see and feel more. Looking outward, we feel our thoughts run away from us. Focusing inward—this takes some disci-pline—we reconnect to ourselves, reaping some of the benefits of sleep while awake. (Or are we more "awake" when sleeping? In a sense, yes: In slumber, our brains go into overdrive.) When the chalkboard is washed clean and the screen fills with Pure Empty (well, not a totally blank screen, in that you're focused on the object of your lust), when you're so consumed in the moment, you begin to plateau, drifting in an erotic trance that comes very close to the fabled meditative nirvana.

The rest of the world bleeds away. The noise quiets. The lights soften. The twitching, convulsing mind sighs to a stop. Bliss!

It sounds lovely. But the chatter of the monkey mind is about as hardwired in me as breathing and the beating of my heart. Cue exercises . . . *get there!*

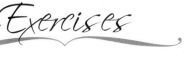

Exercises

1. Submit to the bondage massage. Imagine all your thoughts as picture images and imagine grouping all the pictures together in the center of your forehead. Confine all your thoughts/pictures only to that spot, as if you've collected a roomful of scattered photographs and stacked them into one neat pile, so that you no longer discern individual images but, rather, only a single unit. Hold this particular focus for at least five minutes. Don't strain, but do expend mental effort in maintaining focus on this exercise. I won't tell you what you're likely to feel when doing this exercise. Find it for yourself.

2. Repeat exercise 1 but have your partner engage in verbal role play, projecting his voice from many different locations around your body. Grab each sensual phrase your partner says and paste it like a thought/picture to the center of your forehead. Then have him repeat the verbal play but don't focus on your thoughts. Instead, react naturally to his words, without following the exercise directions. Take quick note of the difference.

3. Try the first exercise while blindfolded, preferably with some bondage, and have your partner sexually stimulate you. Trying not to lose focus of the exercise, imagine each touch as a warming red color that shoots up your spine, perhaps sparking tingling sensations up the spine and through the back of your neck.

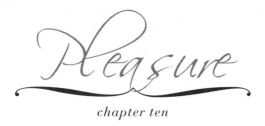

chapter ten

Can you enjoy dominant and submissive role play without inflicting and/or enduring pain? Pain as in actual, real, intense, hurts-the-next-day physical pain? *Mais bien sûr!* Most DSRP does not involve any pain, even playfully delivered. The idea that pain is an essential component of DSRP is a myth used to sell kink trinkets like whips and paddles or whatever Disney twinks toss into their fashion-plate magazine spreads to up their edgy quotient.

Here's the real deal, pumpkin pie: The essence of DSRP is pleasure based on psychological power. Like a Criss Angel Mindfreak escapade, DSRP is pure illusion, kiddo, designed to create and ramp up tension between the sub and dominant. It is lovemaking with a thrilling twist but not always a rough shake. When asked by a male bartender how I like my martini, I say, "Dirty, extra olives, with a twist. I'll do my own shaking, thank you." The barkeep gives me a smirk.

Let's get dirty, twisting, and down with it.

The dominant should sexually tease and frustrate the submissive to induce maximum sexual explosions. Suspense is the key. Withholding is the playbook. It's like the teachings of the *Kama Sutra*, which suggests that one holds off from orgasming for a while, hours even, to achieve one's most powerful orgasm release. That can be very frustrating and maybe feel like torture though the pay-off is the most *wow* release you'll ever have. All good things cum to those who wait . . . a long, long time!

Teasing the submissive sexually not only builds up a powerhaus O. It also helps build the suspense in a scene and gives illusionary power to the dominant over the sub. Once he has his suspense-struck partner under his spell, he's in position to build up the polar play roles of sub and dom—which in turn creates more excitement and heat and tension for both of you. I have found that the more pretend power buildup a dominant is able to muster—or, to put the slipper on the other foot, the more pretend control the sub *loses*—the bigger and better the orgasmic release from your play-induced sexual tension.

By allowing your dom to sexually frustrate you to the twitching brink of madness, you've granted him this accumulation of power. And though the "contractual" ceding of absolute power covers the play period *only*, even a short stint in which the dom holds the reins may work to smooth out knotty kinks in your relationship, thus bringing you pleasure transcending the immediate rewards of one glorious DSRP night. Many self-help books on building healthy relationships claim that a leading cause of "trouble in paradise" tracks to an ongoing power struggle. Commonly, pent-up anger is fought out in a passive-aggressive manner (ask the marriage counselors how fruitful *that* is!). Through DSRP, on the other hand, the partners get a chance to play out that power struggle *openly*. In letting him win—or, in a switch-off, letting yourself win (we discuss switching in chapter 12, "Taboo")—you can defuse the latent resentments of the struggle through scene play. It's amazing what a little exercise of give-and-take, throwing the gripes onto the table, can do to restore equanimity to enemy combatants in a seething battle of the sexes.

A wise man once said that the genius of theater could be seen in that moment at the end of a play when the curtain goes down on a stage littered with dead bodies. A second later, the curtain goes up, and everyone rises to hold hands and take a bow. So is it here. You can play out your power drama without real-life repercussions. You can feel the satisfaction of control or the total abandonment of responsibility in a place where nobody gets hurt.

If the romance is long gone from your relationship (is marital concupiscence an oxymoron?), teasing or being teased—being exquisitely frustrated, or frustrating, to the brink of a squeal—can bring the good times back in a heartbeat. You will feel those first-date jitters of high attraction like they were taking place right now, because they are. Like great "make-up sex" (a line in a novel I read likened it to a pruning), DSRP sexuality is delicious precisely because the partners are letting go of anger, readying themselves for new growth. Usually, this charges up the male, who "rises to the occasion" (ahem) in dominating his woman: a sexy win-win situation for both of you.

When I discovered DSRP I thought, in the prosaic words of that *Fifty Shades* chick, *Holy crap!* This is an amazing medicine for what ails so many personal relationships. Like penicillin arriving in the forties— wow! Exaggeration? Maybe not.

Consider the Small Penis Problem. A small penis can be a big problem for the . . . *female* partner! To judge from the blog posts and the sex manuals, it's tantamount to a world crisis! Well, I'm here to suggest—nay, *insist!*—that DSRP erotic tension building and pleasure techniques can solve the Small Penis Problem. When my girlfriends spill about new loves, they start off with the good stuff—he's sooo great, sooo good looking, sooo charming/funny/smart/witty, blah, blah. Then the Big *But*: *But* he has a small penis. Whereupon they let out a huge sigh of deflation. Hell, I've even noticed that when my friends break up with guys who are physically blessed with a huge cock, they cry a lot harder and longer than when they split with Mr. Uhhhh Shortcoming. It's that hard to let go of a humungo walking vibrator. Really, it is! So, with the small dinky-dick epidemic, what are we to do? Don't lament, kittens, I've got a cure. Sex therapists say the "bad sex from the small penis crisis" is all in *her* mind. Pffft! No. It. Is. *Not.* The girl dating a guy with a little guy wants answers, because, otherwise, speaking frankly, she might as well be dating a cool chick with a big strap-on. *Sighs.* So, here's the drill: Building a scintillating DSRP scene and plunging into the play will spark your nerve endings to a next-level pitch that just doesn't blaze from the dying embers of slobbering-foreplay-then-some-of-the-old-in-'n'-out. It can make you so open and vulnerable, so wildly aroused as to overpower your senses with the illusion that this "new" guy in your life is the Herculean hunk of your dreams. Suddenly, the rapture is overwriting all else in your conscious mind. Suddenly, you have "bigger" things on your mind. What puny penis?

Promises.

Now Let's Put the Play into Play

To heighten sexual pleasure via DSRP, sexual teasing is key, and any man can do it. Even if he's not a great lover, nothing to swoon over in your diary entries. *Sighs.* No worries. We'll turn him into your sex god. It's quite simple, really: just train him, making sure he fully understands the play platform and does what he is told. Ready? Write this word with your reddest red lipstick on his penis and whip him around to look in the mirror: S-L-O-W. Yahaha, I kid, I kid, but the thought is valid, and I'd actually be tempted to do this if I had a wham-bammy boring-speedy lover droning away on top of me with little foreplay or sensuality.

Tell him to play with you extreeeeemely slowly. In this 140-character, ADD-addled culture, you may need to reacquaint him with the concept of slow 'n' easy does it. Undressing you, foreplay, and all the rest must be unhurried and teasing. Think about the popping of a button, the movement of a finger down from that button and encircling the next button . . . this is not time a-wasted, bro—ask any stripper! As said earlier, the built-up orgasm-geyser that this tension creates way, way surpasses the usual hasty bumping of uglies that constitutes vanilla sex as we know it. A given in DSRP is that foreplay should be so slow as to practically torture you, bring you to the point that you're, like, begging him to be allowed to orgasm.

In the first chapter I wrote that most men like a challenge (e.g., sports, hunting, the back-and-forth of business deals). So if he just doesn't get it, or doesn't *want* to get it, try this: Set up a playful challenge for him, the challenge being that he has to try to get you so turned on and panty-soaked that you cannot stand the sexual frustration anymore and are reduced to begging him to bring you to orgasm. *Make him make you beg.* It becomes a sexy little power-play game of who caves in first. You can playfully egg him on with teasing taunts like "I bet you can't make me beg for it." Let's hope you lose.

Below is a small offering of techniques we'd think should "come naturally" to guys looking to maximize the pleasure factor via DSRP, but, uh, maybe not. Let's start sipping that dirty posh martini. Bottoms up!

Slow Foreplay Teasing

I have found this works best when the sub is in light or heavy bondage. The dom should rotate among these three areas.

1. Ear stimulation. Very arousing. Soft pinching, light licking. No slobbering! Ugh.
2. Breasts. Have him spend lots of time pinching, licking, sucking, and all that jazz.
3. The V-area. Lots of clitoral stimulation, with hands, tongue, or vibrator. He can leave one finger inside you and/or circle his finger around the V opening.

As the DSRP trick to bondage foreplay is a slow pace, you may have to tell him when you are close to orgasming so that he knows to pull back with the teasing. Take a time-out and then proceed. Also, he might distract/jolt you by implementing some light pain, e.g., dripping candle wax, applying ice cubes. Other possibilities for enhancing pleasure through light pain are cited in the next chapter. The almost-there moment is also a good time to initiate verbal role play.

Note: DSRP is a spicy/sweet dish. (Spicy is the subject of the next chapter.) If it's all sweet, it's like vanilla sex. If it's all playful pain, the sub's body will become numb and the thrill will be lost. What you need to remember is to tell your dominant to fluctuate back and forth between pleasure and playful, light-stimulus pain. This seesawing keeps the sub's body fully stimulated and pulsing with lightning bolt–level thrills.

Verbal teasing

The gift verbal taunts give to your play scene is one highly valued by the pro-dommes: Teases and commands help to create environments that facilitate both parties' identification with their characters.

Funny, if a guy calls a girl a slut while hanging out, he's in big trouble. If he calls a girl a slut during role play, he scores points. You can teach him which play words you like either by simply spelling things out (being a brave girl) or in giving "reverse" hints during scenes. Barking "I'm *not* a slut" should be a sure invitation to him to drag you through the dirt with just that kind of provocative insult.

Or you might spur him on by half-playfully insulting him. "Get off of me, you pig" should incite him to give it back to you, *verbally*. Verbal play is a mighty potent ingredient in any DSRP scene. Y'know, sticks 'n' stones and all that.

Verbal play doesn't have to be humiliating. Your dominant simply may be very firm in telling you what he wants and expects from you. For example: "You have five seconds to spread your legs for me"; "I want you to bend over this table"; "Crawl to the bathroom and then return in five minutes flat." Verbal play can be as bullying and thrilling—and *pleasuring!*—as any whip, paddle, or kink pain toy, if not more so. Your dominant doesn't have to wield a whip to create the illusion that he's in control and means to capitalize on the power of that position. Language and a commanding tone of voice can do it all, as any good prosecuting attorney can tell you.

The Water Orgasm and Stimulation

If you Google *water pressure orgasm* (bathtub faucet, shower head), you will find a slew of message-board posts and sex articles reporting that a stream of water pressure on your clitoris can deliver one of the best orgasms you will ever have. You might think of it as an "organic" type of stimulation: naturally occurring, harmless, delivering a feeling very unlike the sensation produced by the hands or mouth. Its power is a bit otherworldly (heaven-sent, if you ask me), and if you've never tried it, you soon might find yourself hooked!

Have your dominant take you to the bathroom. You can crawl, he can carry you, he can lead you by your tied-up hands, or he can command you to walk there. Have him command you to spread your legs and position your clitoris directly under the faucet or attachment showerhead. Arch your hips a bit to hit the sweet spot. You can ask him to adjust the heat and pressure of the water. If you have an adjustable, handheld shower faucet, he can control the stream and tease you along to a massive water-gasm. You will be water-jet orgasmed to smithereens and can end your scene there or head back to bed for more traditional orgasms. Use the bathroom as a set, light candles, use scents. To crank it up, he can pull your hair, stimulate your breasts, hold your hands back, or use verbal humiliation, while letting the water work its magic.

Once you are in a state of heavy endorphin-release arousal, your body will be a thousand times more welcoming to some *playful* pain. Light to medium pain will not "hurt" in this aroused state so much as it will provide that spice to the sweetness that makes DSRP an art form.

Warning: To stay in character, you shouldn't take any action until told to do so by your dominant. If you want to move or have your legs untied, take a break, get water, whatever, ask your dominant for permission. Otherwise the illusion of his being in control over you will evaporate!

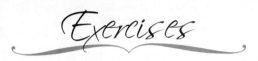

Exercises

1. Grab your iPad or your little black book and put all of the pleasure techniques described and listed in this chapter under one of three categories: "Would try it!" "No way!" "Decide later."

2. Reread your list once a day for a week. Try to set aside a specific time of the day or night to do this, and as you read, try to envision yourself and your fantasy dominant engaged in each activity. It's totally okay if you get stuck on one section and it makes you want to reach for the vibrator. Even better, as this heightens your impatience for that action to be played out, and when it does, you'll be all the more aroused. Make adjustments if you change your mind about swapping categories on any given actions, and be open to adding other actions to the list. At the end of the week, your "Decide later" list may be blank.

3. Show, email, text, fax, or read your full list to your partner. This way he will know: (1) what you want, (2) what you do *not* want, i.e., your hard limits, and (3) what remains on your "maybe" list (do you still have one?)

Now, on to chapter 11 and the element that titillates and (for some) terrifies. We move on to light to medium playful and stimulating "pain." (If we were conversing, those would be air quotes, dahlings!)

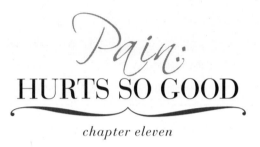

HURTS SO GOOD

chapter eleven

There was a star riding through clouds one night,
and I said to the star, 'Consume me.'
—Virginia Woolf, *The Waves*

What do we talk about when we talk about pain? It's an illusion, you know. Not that we don't see stars when we slam a finger in the car door, say. (&*#$%!!! And that's as *real* as it gets). Rather:

- Pain is illusory: It's not tangible—scientists can't constructively map it, surgeons can't cut it out, moms can't put a Band-Aid on it.
- Pain is a signal: We experience it as a message generated by our nervous system to warn and protect us.
- Pain is subjective: What we experience is personal and unique.
- Pain is relative: The level of pain we feel is a function of our state of mind.

I broach the subject of pain because pain and pleasure are two of our primary motivators, and in this chapter we're going to tread *lightly* into pain-as-pleasure territory—pain that *hurts* but doesn't *harm*, a critical distinction drawn emphatically within these pages.

First off, some thoughts I find interesting, from one of the medical professionals we'd all shun if they didn't stock laughing gas.

While I was visiting my parents, my mother received a call from her dentist. Like a ruthless reporter hot on a case, and recalling that about 25 percent of my dominatrix sessions involved my being asked to role-play a dentist to the sub's "patient," I asked to speak with him regarding the fear of dentists (the phobia has a name, I learned: *odontophobia*) and of the related pain (*algophobia*) and how he handles these common issues with his patients.

I told the dentist that I was doing research on pain. He said that in his experience, patients who are scared and anxious report feeling "substantially greater amounts of pain" than those who are relaxed.

He said that he gives his patients "preps" to relax them, and that, based on his observation and feedback from patients, he has observed that those who are thus prepped experience considerably reduced amounts of pain.

"What preps?" I asked.

"When they first sit in the chair, I tell them to close their eyes and breathe deeply. I explain to them that every procedure I intend to do I will spell out in detail beforehand."

"Why?"

"I have found that fear is the primary cause of most pain. That fear heightens the feeling of pain because anxiety releases adrenaline, which generally makes a person jumpy, easily startled, and unable to relax. By knowing what to expect, a patient's fear is greatly diminished. For people who have extreme fear of the dentist, I tell them to repeat *I am not afraid of the dentist* three times a day for a week before their visit. I have found that helps significantly in reducing pain."

SIGMUND FREUD DREW A DISTINCTION BETWEEN fear and anxiety. Fear, as I interpret his words, is the sensation one might have while walking through the woods and seeing a rattlesnake slither nearby. Anxiety, on the other hand, is the feeling one experiences while walking through the woods thinking, *There's bound to be a snake here . . . I know it . . . or a grizzly bear . . . or a guy with a chainsaw . . .*

Fear, like pain, is an energy pattern in the mind of the perceiver, justifying a "fight or flight response" to an actual threat. But anxiety (as distinct from sensible watchfulness) can elicit that same hormonal response and can provoke the same attendant jumpiness, accelerated heart rate, and elevated blood pressure. Whereas chronically running on such "high alert" has a negative impact on health, a short-term adrenaline rush, such as we experience routinely in the face of the unexpected, can be put to delicious use in DSRP.

To stretch the metaphor a bit: Pain is in the nerve of the beholder. A smack on the arse delivered after moments of anxious dread—when is that menacing, raised arm going to strike the blow?—hurts much more than a spontaneous, playful spank. In other words, the anticipation of a painful blow determines the ouch.

IN MY EXPERIENCE WITH DSRP, THERE are two kinds of pain in play, and they properly belong in separate categories.

PAIN AS PAIN: There are people who enjoy jolts of a stinging sensation, which create a drug-like rush of adrenaline/endorphin exhilaration throughout the body. This is just physical fact, covering a subset of people who, for example, get off on turning the speed on the treadmill up to eleven. Or the yogi who enjoys the painful sensation of stretching his body past his comfort zone, into splits or preposterous pretzels. (Note: I am a *P*-is-for-*playful* disciple of DSRP. I neither engage in nor condone the sort of rough-play DSRP that cripples its practitioners with pain, causes injury, and leaves obvious marks. My counsel to women is leave the "trophy bruises" to the callow high-school footballers and the swaggering "big boys" . . . who really aren't.)

PHANTOM (SYMBOLIC) PAIN: This is of a different stripe. The naughty girl who bends over for a playful spank on the arse is not particularly grooving on the sensation of her screaming arse-nerves. It is the scene, the submission, the humiliation, the *emotion* of the moment that is most important. The pain is not an end in itself but a thing to be gotten through to get to the shiver of the *emotion* of the scene. This makes the pain a sort of supporting player in the scene, a necessary evil, a little meek ow-ie that is part of playing the role. The dominant should execute the actions described below with light force, if the submissive wants— and has signed on for—only *symbolic* pain.

HERE, I INTERJECT SOME THOUGHTS BEFORE moving on to examples. Among the citizenry, there continues to be pervasive fear and moralism pertaining to BDSM. This attitude stems from the misconception that the pain play in BDSM is violent, when, in fact, among the practitioners who believe in the importance of keeping things "safe, sane, and consensual," it is no more violent than a visit to the dentist: the dominant will tell the sub what he is about to do, will proceed slowly, and will back off when the sub uses a safe word. Light to medium pain that does no harm to one's body, in combination with psychological verbal play, sensory deprivation, and bondage, can be as hardcore thrilling as the grievous abuse demanded by extremist devotees. The kinky delights of DSRP, a.k.a. good, clean, erotic fun, may lead to coitus, or they may not, but they should bring catharsis, i.e., the purging of the emotions, something the classic Greek tragedians effected through art, not brutality. I toss out this thought for the record, though I doubt *you* need to hear it; it's unlikely a pain junkie will be drawn to a book of this title.

As pain is relative and as pain thresholds vary, one cannot judge the level of DSRP pain another may find stimulating. A paddle to the behind, for instance, may feel like a love tap to an aroused DSRP sub, while a nonaroused or fearful person may experience that same paddling as a painful, violent hit. Advice to both dom and sub: Do not presume to judge another person's pain threshold, when all you can possibly know is your own. The inflicting of unwelcome pain constitutes abuse.

And one more note: I highly, *highly* recommend sexually pleasurable "sweet teasing" before engaging in any stingy, salty DSRP action. The sweet will feel sweeter when intensified by pain-relieving endorphins. The stings will sting more disagreeably, physically and mentally, if the sub is not first aroused, sexually or otherwise. Think of the health rituals of steam and sauna bathing in such institutions as the Russian and Turkish Baths on the Lower East Side of Manhattan (Frank Sinatra and Timothy Leary were said to have been patrons). The client is advised to start things off by relaxing in the sauna, then run out and dip into a stinging, ice-cold pool, then head back to the sauna, and repeat; the magic, the health benefits, and the thrills are in the artful balance of hot and cold. In European capitals, the ritual is said to involve the swatting of the body with birch branches to stimulate blood circulation. (Those kinky Russkies!—they start out warm and then get icy, spicy, and stingy.) One form of DSRP (which includes some sting) is contrived to mimic the ebb and flow of the ocean waves with an interplay of pleasurable caresses and slight stings to awaken the senses and render a heightened sexual/sensory experience. Think more along the lines of a sexy black rhinestone-headed crop delivering little pings of love taps to your rump, instead of a wicked batch of branches beating your back. Ouch! I'll take the patter of pretty beads, thank you.

Putting the Moves On

Here are some light to medium practices drawn from DSRP's salty department of "pain" . . . to be used as you please. None of these routines, carried out as instructed, will injure or harm the sub's body. We will not be discussing any kink toys, like crops for example, until the last chapter (for advanced practitioners interested in edgier play.)

The art of DSRP playful punishment pain is best performed by a dominant committed to "taking it easy": telling the sub what he is about to do; listening carefully for the sub's safe word and calling a halt when it is uttered. Sexually arousing the sub prior to pain play helps to diminish fear and lessen tension, thereby rendering "pain" more stimulating than hurtful. With the ensuing release of endorphins, the experience becomes wholly pleasurable and spicy. Think fire: It can burn or warm a cold body. The dominant should know that he is playing with fire and proceed accordingly. Read that *very, very carefully*.

Arse Slapping

This can be light and symbolic or heavier for those who enjoy pain as pain. I recommend hand-spanking over paddles, whips, or crops, especially for first-time players, because it's almost impossible to do any harm in spanking with an open hand. (In fact, there's a good chance the dominant's hand will begin to sting and hurt well before the sub's arse does!) Curiously, cupping the hand while arse-spanking increases the illusion of pain while decreasing the sting. Cupping results in the shock of a louder sound, which will heighten the sensory input, conveying to the sub that the slaps are heavier and more powerful than they actually are. Blows from a cupped hand, however, are in fact physically less "punishing."

Hair Pulling or Grabbing

This causes only phantom pain if done correctly. I'm not talking about hair pulling street-fight style. Nooo, not sexy! An aggressive, fast, and sloppy yank by the dominant is guaranteed to piss you off. The way it should be done, and you should so instruct your dominant, is for him to place his palm on the back of your neck, spread his fingers through your hair, grab a huge chunk of hair in his fist, and draw back firmly. The larger the chunk, the more stimulating and less painful it will be. If, in your play agreement, you agree to some hair pulling yet fail to show him how it's done, you will regret it. It will hurt you, make you furious, hurt his feelings, spoil the moment, and set the scene for a later fight erupting from your pent-up resentment. It can also wreck a perfectly lovely evening.

Face Slapping

This qualifies as phantom or slightly stingy pain as pain. Okay, this is best done quickly and with spirit. A sharp, "Hey, wake up!" slap is far less aggressive and painful than a slow and heavy one. Think raindrops hitting your window in quick little tap-tap-taps, not the rock-hard, steady pound of hailstones. The dominant should always aim for the cheek, never, ever the ear or lips. This is a good attention-getting stimulus for raising the endorphin levels, if the sub is extremely sexually aroused. It can provide a welcome blood rush and signal the promise of exciting things to come, if done spontaneously and with authority. Face slapping is most potent and best received right after delivery of a rousingly pleasurable sexual act performed on the sub or during feel-good penetration.

V/Body Slapping

This can cause phantom or light to medium pain as pain. It can be done slow or fast with light to medium force—*no heavy hitting here!* Not because I'm a Debbie Downer prude but because the more forceful the slap, the sharper the pain and the more numbing to the sub's erogenous zones. Overdo it, and soon she will feel no pain or pleasure. Not so hot, right? Right. The art here is to stimulate the V area, not to knock it out of commission. Also, vagina slapping remains a primal taboo because that area is the most sensitive on a woman's body. V slapping instantly can create delish, overwhelming illusions that your dominant is mighty, powerful, and sexy. As former Secretary of State Henry Kissinger famously said, "Power is the ultimate aphrodisiac," and, as I see it, there may be no truer truism. In one study, in which women were asked to choose between a movie star and a president of the United States, the majority chose POTUS. Power does it for women. Youth is sexy to men.

Just how it is. Birds and bees, guys . . . whatcha gonna do? It's how we're wired, and V slapping plays into that, inducing through body language the feeling that he is laying claim, announcing to the world, "This V is mine! I claim it! Roar!" His desire for you will heighten yours for him, and vice versa.

Nipple Pinching

This can cause phantom or light to medium pain as pain. Yes, there are nipple clamps, but I've rarely seen a male or female sub tolerate nipple clamps for more than five minutes before they become painful and annoying. (Clamps, after all, do torture us into de Sade territory.) Also, in my experience, subs find the human touch much more erotic and physiologically powerful than some cold toy. I acknowledge, however, that there are people who find toys exciting—yeah, yeah, I've heard Rihanna belt out "chains and whips excite me"—so okay, I've got you covered in the last chapter. Just to let you know, though, I won't be discussing blood or heavy pain. Posh home girl don't play that game. Your dominant can use nipple pinching to inflict light pain as a way to force you into doing what he wants, threatening not to release you until you do this or that. If you're interested in exploring this, I'd suggest talking about it beforehand or being prepared to use your safe word or action to let him know to back off and unhand (or unclamp).

I REMAIN AN ADHERENT OF PLAYFUL pain actions (whether they involve phantom/symbolic pain or pain as pain) that the dominant may employ to enhance the sweetness of pleasure. Such activities heighten endorphin release and confuse the body, signaling a speed-up, slow-down, or whatever it takes to awaken your senses for maximum enlivened sexual pleasure. The more endorphins, the better the orgasm, the more endorphins. Ahhh. Sweet, sweet love taps. *Merci*, lover.

Exercises

1. Do a yoga or other tendon-stretching workout. Find the tipping point where your body begins to transmit the onset of low, numbing pain, signaled as more a euphoric rush of salty pings than "hurt," which is a clear warning that you have pushed your body too far. (This point will be different for everyone—to each according to her own pain threshold.) At that moment, just as the spicy/sweet spot threatens to tip into "shit, this *hurts*!" territory, you're *there*! You've met the sensation you're going to feel in your spicy play, should you decide to play on the pain side. Store the memory of that moment of exhilarating release, and use it to gauge the level of pleasure/pain you're experiencing in your DSRP. *Do not* allow yourself to go past that point. Awwwright, you're thinking I'm a Debbie Downer, while you're gearing up to crack the whip, go all the way, *and* be cool with it. My POV is this: If the play hurts, then (1) you are unlikely to continue and you'll likely flip out if your partner storms out after you have "suffered for him," and (2) you risk getting dangerously addicted to the pain, wanting more and more till your body needs to be ripped up to satisfy your addiction. I've seen this happen with subs in the scene, and it's ugly. It's not DSRP, it's S&M.

2. Before you and your partner try any spicy DRSP, first try every toy and action on yourself. Yeah, I know, I'm thinking the same thing: "Who the hell is going to crop her own arse alone in the living room?" Well, if you want to have a smooth play scene, you'll do just that. Mr. H refuses to play with anyone new to DSRP who doesn't confirm that she's first tested out the gags, crops, etc., on herself. Nothing is guaranteed to kill a scene like a freak-out during play, when you realize your eyes were bigger than your stomach, so to speak. Do test-drive the equipment, so you don't end up in the backseat of the car with no directions for the driver.

3. As in the first exercise in chapter 10, grab your iPad or your little black book and enter or list all of the punishing actions, verbal and physical, sweet and salty, described in this chapter under one of three categories: "Would try it!" "No way!" "Decide later." If you don't want to show the list to your partner, you must spell out to him what you want and what is unacceptable to you in punishment play. If he's a newbie, it may be a good idea to dig up an online BDSM video that highlights an item from your "want" list and let him see the moves in action.

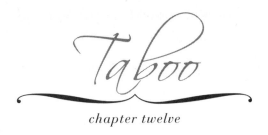

chapter twelve

Frances: Besides, I don't want to be what you want to make me.
Dr. Symington: And what's that?
Frances: Dull. Average. Norrrr-mal.
—*FRANCES* (1982), STARRING JESSICA LANGE

This exchange, which takes place between Frances Farmer, the head-strong actress of the thirties and forties, and the chief psychiatrist at the mental institution where she has been involuntarily committed, captures all the spirit and doom-courting of the gorgeous, talented actress, an early supporter of feminist causes. Farmer's fractious personality kept her in perpetual hot water with the chauvinistic studio bosses. Still, if playing it normal means always acting the Obedient Good Girl, accepting the stripping of one's individuality—kinky quirks and all—then I'm with Frances. And, yes, I read her autobio, and I know things didn't turn out well. But her assertiveness in the face of authoritarianism (never thought I'd find a place to use that ten-buck word), and her fierce fight for her identity and independence, seem perfectly suited to a chapter playfully named "Taboo."

"We're Kinky, Not Crazy"

Criticizing the inclusion of "paraphilic disorders" in the fifth edition (2013) of the *Diagnostic and Statistical Manual of Mental Disorders*, writer Jillian Keenan, in an online post, argues that it is "unscientific, and stigmatizing."[1] Keenan quotes a sexologist who defines the condition of "paraphilia" as having "unusual sexual interests," and she clarifies that these include "sexual masochism disorder, fetishistic disorder, transvestic disorder, and so on." I've cited Ms. Keenan's article in the endnotes, as you may wish to read her essay in full. It's worth it, as her points are well taken. For our purposes, the situation may be summarized in her own words: "Simply put, the *DSM V* will say that happy kinksters don't have a mental disorder. But unhappy kinksters do. . . . To be diagnosed with one of these noncriminal sexual disorders, the person must 'feel personal distress about their interest.'"

Huh? Are you thinking what I'm thinking? What about those folks distressed over other esoteric interests, e.g., bird-watching (uh oh, am I eccentric?), ballroom dancing (uh oh, too fey?)? More pertinently, homosexuality used to be defined as a disorder if it caused personal distress; the idea that the distress might be rooted in society's treatment of homosexuals rather than in the orientation itself doesn't seem to have occurred to the writers of the *DSM*. That the classification of a disorder is based on having qualms strikes me as facile, arbitrary, and just plain silly. Paraphrasing a friend's post to my Facebook account: With the American Psychiatric Association accepted as the official arbiter in defining normality, what about those experimenting with DSRP for the first time, finding themselves in a high state of anxiety because of socially induced shame? According to this latest reading of "mental disorder," are they, too, to be regarded as being in need of treatment? My friend's reaction was something on the order of: hogwash. Publicly, I stand with him, even as I prepare to discuss the heavier side (some may say the "dark side," and I won't argue the point) of DSRP, which may be what the APA means to relegate to the treatable-disorder category. Even so, I prefer that sexologist's term, *unusual* (as having red hair is unusual), to describe the interest in heavier kink practices, as I see it as neither a mental disorder nor harmful, if all activities are consensual and played according to *humane*, precontracted rules. (I know a few heavy-hitters, and while I don't share their affection for extreme play, I find them no crazier than the butcher, the baker, or my third-grade teacher.)

There are kink-friendly psychiatrists who happily accept their patients' kinky lifestyles, though their professional outlook is hardly mainstream. None of them, I wager, would have sided with Frances Farmer's Hollywood studio bosses who were complicit in shipping her off to the psych ward: OMG, such an *unruly* woman, such *strong* opinions, such *fight* . . . def a danger to society!

Advanced Kink

There's a reason I've saved this material to wind things up. Well, actually two reasons: First, I've included some extreme practices that belong at the far edge (but not the farthest) of kink and DSRP—beyond my chosen play territory—and second, I wanted to be able to issue a content warning to qualmish readers (with assurances that no one's going to call them "dull, average, normal" if they're not interested in reading this material), so they may know to skip this chapter and move on to the kink bazaar source guide to DSRP-related films, books, and products in the appendix.

As first mentioned in chapter 3, a central, but very dangerous component of advanced DSRP is edge play. You might think of edge play as standing-on-the-edge-of-a-cliff-without-a-bungee-cord edgy. It can be dangerous to the mental and physical health of a devil-may-care submissive who hasn't proper appreciation for the dangers. Submissive aficionados engage in edge play because they find it a racy and thrilling delight. Playing "on the edge" presupposes that the sub and the dominant have agreed that the dominant can do *whatever he wants* to the sub at *any time* during playtime. For lifestyle edge players, that license is extended to anytime, period. The sub has set *no* limits, and not because she's okay with a fractured skull or a whip-savaged face (explained straightaway). I do not recommend edge play to anyone new to DSRP, who hasn't been practicing, let's say, for at least a year *with the same partner.* This helps ensure that you will be able to trust your dominant to know your unspoken limits, your likes and dislikes, and to refrain from pushing you too far. If he does—and I address this to those who might be thinking, "I don't care, I love it/him so, so much"—get away from him *immediately.* Overstepping humane bounds plunges into unhealthy sadist and masochist (BDSM or S&M) territory. It is not what DSRP is about and not what this book is about and nothing I endorse, here or elsewhere. Heavier edge players may send me finger-wagging hate mail, but that's my uncompromising stand, my *limit,* if you will, and besides, *The Posh Girl's Guide* wasn't written for them.

Another central component of advanced DSRP is play that involves pain for pain's sake. Okay, I gotta come clean here. Yes, yes, I admit that in my time as a dominatrix I was happy to administer extreme pain to the male subs who begged for it and *loved* it—pain sluts, as they're nicknamed within the scene. I'm not a timid person; I thrive on adventure and the unknown. Whipping and paddling men till they bleed? I found their need intriguing. Kicking men in the balls I also found interesting. I even helped brand one sub, holding the blowtorch while another mistress put the branding iron into the blue flame and branded the happy sub's arse. All these pain slut subs were *addicted* to heavy pain.

I since have changed my mind about withholding judgment on subs who like and demand heavy pain. Any action that causes the body to be heavily bruised or bloodied—such is the aftermath of multiple kicks to the vulnerable testicles, for example—I now would refuse to carry out. No longer neutral on the subject, I consider those who demand such excessive and hazardous treatment as being dangerously addicted to pain because, as I've seen, their demands for more and more punishing severity escalate as, apparently, their tolerance of pain is hiked. Their pain habit grows, exactly as the junkie craves ever-increasing dosages of body-wasting drugs. Apart from my compunctions about the dangers to mental and physical health posed by such extreme practices, I contend that tissue-bruising, blood-letting, and the like are not necessary components of enjoyable kink activity. Sure, people elect to get body modifications—tattoos, heavy piecing, breast implants, nose jobs—but few are driven to obsession, and when they are, we see it as troubling, alarming. Who wasn't thinking, "Eeeek, what derelict butcher would allow Michael Jackson to undergo all those deforming nose jobs?" If you do insist on play with heavy pain, try to limit yourself to the rare occasion, sorta like a treat, so you don't end up on the hamster wheel of serious hurt, requiring more extreme pain to *feel* anything. The point of role play, even in the extreme, is not to desensitize or numb or condition or *harm* the body but to excite, awaken, and free it. So with that said, here's a list of toys designed to cause medium to heavy pain. Proceed with caution and take it slow 'n' easy.

Tapping and Other Pain Toys for Use in Play

Floggers

A flogger is a handle with many ribbons. The wider the strip, the less sting it causes. It is possible to deliver a light flogging, which feels like "a thousand fingers touching you at once," according to my sub friend Aaron Edelman. Heavy flogging is much safer than whipping, caning, or cropping. Have your dominant Google-search for free videos on the various ways to use the flogger. Many floggers are made of leather, but you can opt for a fur or soft-tail flogger instead. Obviously very safe, these offer a sensation that really does feel like love taps and deliver no sting.

Crops

The iconic instrument of dominance. These are very safe sting toys. It's easy to go light with a crop, as it takes a lot of arm power to go hard, unlike the toys detailed below. You can buy crops for less than $25 at any kink store. You can also find glam, $500 rhinestone-headed models at AgentProvocateur.com, as mentioned in my appendix shopping list. There's even a model that folds up to tuck discreetly into a lady's handbag. *Shhhh!*

Paddles

Another DSRP icon. Paddles fit cozily into a "punishment" play scene or naughty girl scene, for the sub who wants to explore salty actions. You wouldn't expect it, but wooden paddles sting much less than leather ones. Any "whack" kink toy that is flexible creates more sting. Among leather paddles, hard leather behaves more like a wooden paddle, for safer sting play, whereas a leather flap, not stiff, gives a more slapping sting.

Single-tail Whips

Uhh, really not a good idea, unless you have been playing for at least a year, have read up on single-tails, and have watched some instructional kink videos. They are potentially dangerous for both the sub and the dom. Once, when I was using a single-tail whip on a male sub, the whip recoiled and lashed me across the eye socket. Fun, huh? Well, they can be, if you are very experienced in handling them. Dominatrices I knew practiced hours a day. I suggest having the dominant practice using the whip on pillows and target marks on walls to perfect his aim and force-control. Start with a whip three to four feet in length. Do *not* buy a longer one until you master this length. Vendors sell whips longer than four feet but they're used more for kink party "shows" and other non-kink exhibitions like Annie Oakley's Wild West Show. Rule of thumb: The longer the whip, the harder it is to control and master. Be warned. My advice remains: Do not go down this road.

Cat o' Nine Tails

This is a multi-tailed whip, like a combo flogger and single-tail. It is a dangerous toy in inexperienced hands.

Nipple Clamps

Buy only the rubber-coated ones, not metal. When your dominant is putting them on or removing them, he should do so very gently and slowly. During play, it's okay for him to tug on them a bit, but not too hard and never, ever fast.

Canes

For disciplining naughty British schoolboys, Catholic schoolgirls (ancient history, I must interject), and now, well, for fun! The thicker the cane, the less velocity, potency, and sting. This isn't to say that thick canes can't pack a wallop, and I would recommend them. The thin ones can slice. Eeek! No one needs that.

red flag! red flag! getting into heavy territory!
ATTENTION MUST BE PAID!

Electric Play (quadruple eeeks)

There is a power box made by ErosTek that comes with tons of attachments, ranging from electric pulsating dildos to gloves and clamps that work like electroshock clothespins to lightly clutch the body and deliver a charge. Hunt around in the "electric" sections of the kink stores for other toys. Do not use an electric device without first reading through the directions and being sure you understand them. Better yet, have an experienced player or kink store employee explain it to you in person.

Okay, Enough Spice, It's Sexy Time, Kittens

Practices and tools of edge DSRP may involve advanced pain, or advanced pleasure, as you dictate.

Vibrators and Dildos

There are models that simultaneously stimulate the clitoris and inside the V—the double-headed lover. During play, I would stay away from too much overpowering stimulation such as delivered by this model, as you are more likely to orgasm quickly and kill the sexy buildup of the DSRP scene. If your partner uses the double stimulator, I would suggest using it in small, thirty-second spurts (ha).

SILICONE: Buy silicone *everything* rather than rubber. It is much smoother and feels better (and has no rubbery odor).

METAL: The websites listed in the appendix offer metal dildos, vibrators, and even, I see, anal plugs. It might appear gimmicky but it's said to bring an entirely new material sensation to your body, adding more mental and physical stimulus. Also, metal feels more intensely commanding. (You *will* pay attention!)

WITH KNOBS FOR EXTRA STIMULATION: There are vibrators and dildos with little candy-colored knobs that are said to add extra V friction and, hence, stimulation. Honestly, I've never tried one, so I can't advise you to def spend your mad money on this one, but I've heard a few friends rave about them with eye-rolling drama. Whatevs.

ELECTRIC (FOR THE V OR BACKDOOR AREAS): Yep! 2013. We have that ErosTek control panel with knobs that ramp up the shocks, from very light and fuzzy to a more zinging zap. Electricity sounds frickin' terrifying, I know, but hear me out, players. Electric play can double the pleasure in that it's adding extra waves of stimulating vibration. Yes, yes, you can regulate to create pleasurable or stingy-shocky sensations—just don't turn up that dial too far! They even sell anal plugs that attach to the panel to expand and contract the pegs for pulsing action. You could use it for the V area, as well. I've never tried it, only because I'm not a shopper and neither am I really into toys for personal play, but it sounds like a home run to me! Furthermore, it gathers rave reviews.

iPod-triggered (there's an app for that?): Also on the kink store menu are vibrators you can sync to your iPod—get this! The damn thing pulses to the rhythm of the music! A little gimmicky for me but maybe sounds groovy to you?

Feather ticklers

Well, you can always use the duster, but if you want something a bit more chichi, stores offer feather ticklers that are great for, yeah, tickling. Said to be great for soothing and calming the body after an arse paddling or other salty action.

Fur gloves

Fantastic for calming the nerves and reducing adrenaline levels after any salty "pain" actions, from nipple pinching to arse whipping. As a dominatrix, I always used a fur glove to stroke my sub's pain areas immediately after inflicting pain. My subs would instantly relax and tone down. It's also a perfect way to deliver a physical "I'm sorry" to the sub, if the dominant has by accident gone a little past the sub's comfort level. Fur has a very primal, comforting feeling to it. For the PETA gang, there are faux fur gloves.

Anal plug

I have never tried one but from what I gather, they fall out a lot, which is very annoying during a play scene, and they're uncomfortably large. Best, then, to use fingers or a slim vibrator if you want to play in that backdoor area. Ummm, there it is.

Role-Play Extras

These play toys fall under the objectification category. They're used in scenes where the sub happily acts a humiliating role such as an object, a lowborn animal, or something that feels subhuman. Subs report that playing such abject roles furthers the sense of full submission into sub space (described in chapter 4) and that this can feel quite liberating. It's not for everyone, but here 'tis:

Dog Collars

In my domme sessions, standing in front of a businessman-client dressed in a bespoke powerhaus suit with a big-bucks briefcase to match, I could see that it was hard for him to make that instant transition from CEO to my lowly slave. I discovered this trick: If I put a dog collar on the sub as soon as he entered my dungeon, his transformation (in his mind and mine, as well) from boss to slave was instantaneous. I think you'll find, too, that almost nothing beats collaring for ripping the reality rug out from under, leaving a sub on all fours and begging to serve. You can find cheapo spiky collars at any sex or kink store and more elegant ones, some studded with diamonds, on kink couture and luxe lingerie websites. If you're after the real deal, check out the couture fashion lines that sell actual dog collars for the pooches of the posh and famous. Add a leash and off you go like a prize pedigree poodle to sub playland.

Dog Bowls

Having your dominant order you to eat or lap up water (or tiny licks of Champagne) from a dog bowl can intensify the feeling of inhabiting sub-space. Too, if you (the sub) are having a hard time getting into or feeling the role, this can be a helpful trick to hasten the process. It's not for me, but you might dig it!

Open-mouth Gag

Another beastly accessory, this is a metal ring that forces the mouth to stay wide open. It sure adds token muscle to a dom's efforts to produce a "helpless little me" for staging captive scenes. You can find a large assortment of such gags on the kink store websites. I wouldn't recommend them for first-timers, or for anyone who has never played with any sort of mouth gag.

Pony Play

Okay, there are kinksters who are into what is called "pony play." They use a gag designed to look and function like a horse's bit and bridle. And it gets crazier, with gear like human saddles, bits, grooming tools, and anal plugs trailing fake horse tails. There are even human/pony play stable establishments that host such players. Yeah, this is way off the play map for me, but if you've seen the film *Secretary*, you've watched as a saddled-up Maggie Gyllenhaal clearly dug it. To each her own fetish fix.

Chastity Belt

For the faithful maiden awaiting the return of her shining knight, how about the leather chastity belt, with key, to be held by Sir Dom, natch? Not putting total trust in her vows of fidelity, he uses the medieval contrivance to ensure steadfastness, barring her sexual pleasuring till he decides to give it. Google *female chastity devices*. For ye olde times' sake.

Traa-laa-laa-ing away into Heavy Play . . .

Racial Role Play

Always a loaded proposition. I know some dominatrices who refuse to accept requests for racial role play, even when begged by submissives who feel it is not the domme's place to judge. I chose to allow my subs to do the decision making. In fact, I know an African American sub, a man I consider very well rounded and stable, who said he felt deeply offended that his dominatrix refused to do a racial-based role-play scene with him. He said he considered her refusal to constitute reverse racism, more personally insulting than the suggested role play would have been. I can see his point. Now, if you want to try a racial role play, you had better think long and hard, and if you have any misgivings before or during play, stop it immediately, just as you would physical pain play.

Age Play

Awwwright then. A preppy player friend recently wrote to me, speaking of age play: "Like, everyone does it or fantasizes about it. You need to put it in your book. Women are bolted, electrified, by that scene, because giving vent to their daddy fantasy issues is exhilarating precisely *because* it's forbidden." I think she must be right. I really swear to God, I can't think of a single girlfriend who hasn't admitted to being a bit turned on by step-daddy- or daddy-figure-role play, actual or fantasy. And not just my girlfriends. Sooo many stories and little black book secrets from women, all demographics, about entertaining and indulging the . . . let's call it the father figure fantasy and forget Mr. O Complex. One woman, an accomplished PR agent, told Mr. H that she had begun engaging in age play with a BF. She threw out sample scene fare like, "If I'm good, Daddy lets me have a puff of his cigar while I'm tied up." This woman is a smart, savvy, kick-ass businesswoman who eats rival businessmen for breakfast. Also, what to make of young women who dress up in school-girl and cheerleader outfits—"just for amusement"—in the non-kink world? I'd venture that they're entertaining age-play fantasies, and I'd suggest that they indulge, not fret about it.

Google up *daddy sexual fantasy* and you'll find a blue million pages on the subject and learn just how many women share this fancy. So let's talk about it? Haul it out of the shaming taboo shadows of the creepy-creep backwoods and into the sunlight of the *play*ground. The psychology behind it—Oedipal? not incestuous but infantilizing, sugar-daddy-ish?—is not that interesting to me. What *is* interesting is why we can't just "get on with it" and indulge the father figure scene as a fun *fantasy*. Well, we can. Here. And here goes.

The Daddy Deal in Action

1. Your dominant can assume verbal and physical (via props) aspects of a daddy figure who isn't *your* daddy. He can puff on a cigar and let you, if you are a "good girl," take a puff or two (but don't tell Mommy!)

or allow you a sip of his Scotch. You might both be in costume, he in a grown up suit and tie, you in a plaid schoolgirl jumper with knee socks. He might address you as "bad little girl" and give a now-that's-more-like-it nod when you reply, "Yes, sir." These moves imply an age gap, whether or not you've decided to call him "Daddy." With hints, you can skirt the "incest-y" issue.

2. Into exploring full-on incest-y PLAY? (I've used caps as a reminder: We're *playing* here.) Brava! Let's do it! I'd move into the scene slowly and stir up some sexy urges before introducing any "improper" daddy/daughter verbal play. You don't need a psych degree to figure out the attraction of this popular fantasy: Most of us grow up seeing Daddy as a towering symbol of dominance and control, so we should have little trouble transferring our awe and our approval-seeking conduct to a role-playing stand-in. If real Dad was a loving, nurturing parent, I imagine the attitude will be reverential, whereas the daughter of a no-goodski dad may feel and playact as if she's ceding control back to a fearsome sovereign, who, nevertheless, she continues to wish to please. Funny, most of my male subs asked for role play with a *wicked* mommy dearest. Conversely, among the female pros—those tough-talking, hard-ass Amazonian dom-inatrices—locker-room confessions ran to fawning, adoring role-play fantasies explored with their boyfriends. They kept this all hush-hush, of course, lest their male submissives discover the "kink in the armor"—that their dommes entertained sub fantasies of their own, that is. So it swings both ways. *Wink.*

Hey, both of the sexy, hip, smart editors at girls-get-real-and-deal-with-it website xoJane.com, have bravely expressed personal sexual "daddy slash step-daddy" play fantasies in recent articles. It's 2013 and the women at xoJane are telling us the gritty eekie truth (or, at least, their gritty eekie truth), like it or not. That has sparked confessional responses from many of their females commenters, who daily post "me toos!"

Jeez, I and most of my confidants on occasion call up the command-ing father figure, a take-me-by-force fantasy picture splashing across our consciousness during masturbation, or rising from our subconscious in beta-state-of-mind dream sleep. If it's an overriding fantasy that you can't or don't wish to shake off, then go for it on the safe playing field of DSRP. Reluctance stemming from social conditioning may make you more childish than pretending to be one. Was that bitchy? Well, there it is. As I see it.

Oh, Jesus, Mary, and Joseph, what next?

Yep, the Rape Fantasy

Traa-laa-laa. Another hushed-up, masturbating-under-the-sheets fantasy. Where to draw the line? So long as you're operating in fantasy land, I'd say that's up to you. Don't let any male lover tell you that your fantasy is sick.

I here will interject a collateral tale of a cautionary nature, to remind you that you just never do know where your fantasies will take you. This story belongs not to me but to Annie Sprinkle, the *über*-famous porn star (and active feminist). I've been a fan of hers for decades. In the eighties, my mother worked at an ad agency where she struck up a friendship with the artist H. R. Giger's agent, a co-worker of hers. One day, when I was visiting Mom at work (she had her own company, by that time), the agent introduced me to his friend, Annie. She had graduated first in her class at the prestigious School of Visual Arts in New York City and become one of the most popular adult-film stars (and, later, performance artists) of the eighties. Mom had put me to work on an alphabetical sorting project, and I was using tricks to compensate for my dyslexia. Annie knowingly picked up on the cue-card routine, leaned down, and in a motherly tone of voice, said, "Don't worry, sweetie, I'm dyslexic too and look at me now!" (My mother did a silent "Eeeeeeeek!" Ha!)

Anyway, Annie's strong feminist POV was expressed in full in a one-woman show she did years later at PS 122, the performance art space in New York City. She showed clips of her porn movies, shared insights, and, after the show, invited audience members up to the stage to touch her, in whichever way they wished. What was stunning to me (this was in 1998, before the xoJaners started up), Annie admitted (in public!) to once having had continual rape fantasies. She recounted having been deliriously excited over an offer, early in her porn film career, to do a "gang rape" movie. She showed a clip of it and admitted that on set things had turned scary and a bit ugly-real-intense for her. Yes, she could have stopped the "gang rape," but it *was* faux, and, as a pro, she hung in there. The revelation in her spill was that she never again experienced a rape fantasy.

So, heeding what I think was Annie's warning, I'd advise against booking a full-force, gang-rape role-play scene, or even a solo rape-play scene with your partner. Even in a play scenario, things can veer out of control. This presents risks on two fronts: First, and most importantly, you may be injured, and second, you may be squandering a perfectly good fantasy!

If you do go for it, I suggest going slow and taking things in stages, having him first just pin down your arms, nothing more aggro than that. Too, play will be safer with you in verbal command, instructing scene by scene: "Pin my arms, I'm going to struggle, grab my hair." That way, the scene is less likely to swerve into edge play. Absolutely do not set up a fantasy rape date in which your partner calls the shots and, unwittingly perhaps, overwhelms you physically and emotionally.

Lifestyle Kink Beyond the Saturday Night Special

You can delve deeper into the psychological control games, practicing them in extended daily routine. Remember the scene from the previously cited, erotically unorthodox *Secretary* (it's in our appendix "must see" list), with James Spader and Maggie Gyllenhaal, in which she suggests a committed, 24/7, S&M role-play relationship? He, the instigator of it all, sputters, "But we can't live *this* way all the time!" His response was unpredictable, making it a memorable movie moment, and no one who saw it is likely to forget her frank, chipper answer: "Why not?" Why not, indeed! They lived happily ever after! A rhetorical question: Notwithstanding the S&M role play, did any of you really fear for Maggie/Lee's safety with Spader/Mr. Grey? (What the hell is it with these dominating Mr. Greys, anyway?!) Smile . . . I thought not.

Play as Lifestyle

Some kinkster couples draw up submissive/dominant contracts wherein the sub agrees to be the "property" of the dominant. Such couples live a lifestyle of extended role play. I can't imagine signing on to such an agreement, and neither can I imagine it working unless the pair is married or in a serious long-term relationship. Otherwise, diving in this deep, how does one feel if she's left by her dom? I should think it would be along the lines of "I gave you *every*thing and let you do *any*thing and you *leave* me?!" I can see how, within a committed relationship, such an arrangement might create strong bonds, but still, think about the resentment and pain the sub, and perhaps even the dom, would experience should such an intense kink relationship be ripped apart. Not likely to be just another no-fault divorce action.

Outdoor/Public

You can extend your private play to public settings within everyday life, discreetly if that suits, of course. You can engage in role play, in whispers, at restaurants, parties, and public outings. Take hints from *Secretary* and *9½ Weeks.*

Bringing Another Partner into the Play Arena

Warning, though I hardly think it necessary: A kinky threesome, like any other threesome, is verging into treacherous territory, can be very damaging, and can destroy relationships. I wouldn't sign on to such an arrangement, in or out of the kink scene. Based on experiences with threesomes related to me by trio players, I'd say that if you guys decide to try it, both partners should take a long, introspective look at their psychological suitability to the proposition. Also, I like the suggestion that the third party be someone you're highly unlikely to run into again, as in, not a friend or co-worker, not the waitress at your favorite restaurant, etc. The third party should be comfortable with the prospect of the engagement's being a one-time deal—and *that* to be determined by the partners, in the event the threesome play puts unforeseen emotional strain on your relationship. (What's your history with jealousy?) Also, and this might be the most important slice of advice: All parties to the initial playdate should be forewarned and agree that any one of the participants can call a halt at any time, even before play is initiated. Each must understand that this is an experiment that can easily combust, thus justifying carefully planned precautions. Final word: Do *not* get coaxed or seduced into a threesome; nor should you attempt to coax a reluctant partner. Your life/relationship isn't a racy HBO show that you can rewind, so best not to "try out" a threesome on a whim.

THEN AGAIN, TO GIVE YOU A sense of the potential excitement of a threesome, here's a story from Mr. H's files, for the advanced class.

A KINKY THREESOME

She was a sexy, rich, preppy career girl who owned the entire top floor of a tony building in a tony neighborhood of Manhattan. Ever so bored, she longed to up the kink ante. A double-decker this time. In the past, she had allowed Mr. H to use her humungo apartment for his kink trysts with other women—with a catch. Her requirement had been that, during play, he take a picture of the girl, bound but faceless, and then email the pix to her. What use she planned for the photos, she wouldn't say. But that was the deal, and it factored into his decision making in considering her new proposition. Before he indulged her in that proposition—a *ménage à trois* bondage scene with her best friend—he insisted that they all meet at least three times to discuss the details. One girl expressed a wish to be captured by a thuggish mugger. The other said she wanted to discover an intruder in her home and be "taken" by him. Two separate scenes that must occur simultaneously. How to please both? Determined to devise the perfect scene, he painted scenarios and, like a human lie detector, he watched the women for telltale expressions: icked out or bring it on? He didn't suspect the two had ever engaged in bisexual conduct, but he knew they were very close. That knowledge he would use as his hook to surprise them with a nerve-jangling end to the night.

All went smashingly well the night of the big event in her penthouse kink pad. Here's what happened. *Shhhh!* His Hitchcock-kink-ian brain had sniper-targeted the perfect setup. He'd planned that the apartment owner would be at home, while the other exited the elevator and approached her friend's door. He grabbed the visitor in the hallway and "forced" her into the apartment (he had a key), where he tied her up at a far end of the floor. Across the spacious L-shaped room, the other girl awaited her intruder. "Oh, dear! He intruded," she gasped melodramatically as he carried her into her bedroom, threw her forcefully onto the bed, and tied her up. Both girls now were heavily bound, separated from each other's view on opposite sides of the floor. Arms, legs and, oh!, gagged with each other's panties. He was a meanie, a panty-wetting meanie. *Shhhh!* He slipped back and forth from end to end like a smooth cat burglar, sexually teasing one, then returning to titillate the other . . . till it was time. He could tell that the hallway girl was ready. He lifted up the bound damsel and carried her across many rooms to the master bedroom where the mistress of the house lay bound and sexually frustrated. With both girls tied and gagged, he tossed the visitor onto the bed next to the home-invasion victim. Mr. H said he made violent love to her for an hour, as the other watched. I asked why, because she wanted to watch? No, he said, the role-play script was written as a burglary/rape scene in which one girl was forced to watch what was "in store" for her. "Oh," I said, thinking to myself, *He is deliciously evil.* La de da, yes, please.

Annnnd, it got worse! *Wink.* He switched targets, leaving the first girl bound, panting, and satisfied. When he moved for the switch, the mistress of the house was shaken from having witnessed his manhandling and verbal humiliation of the first victim. Like a boorish brute, he'd called her "my first slut of the night," which had been a marvelous turn-on. Mr. H knew it would take a lot to un-bore the ennui-afflicted mistress of the house, and he knew exactly how to do it. Wide-eyed and quivering, she sank into the bed under his six-foot-four frame, as he sank into her—commanding her love, to put a polite spin on things. It ended with her room-shaking meowings of pleasure.

But . . . this was not to be the final act, as the women were expecting. Already bound and helpless, they were now arranged into sexually humiliating positions, one girl's face very close but not touching the other girl's . . . well, we'll dredge up an old locution and just call it the sixty-nine position. The girls were stirred by rage, spewing plumes of sexual shockwaves into the room. After a suitable cooling-down period, he untied them, gave a Zorro-like adieu-to-all-that, kissed their hands, and, like a gentleman, exited stage left. Poof! Leaving behind a trail of red-hot fairy-tale dust, he was gone.

The next day, Mr. H received a text from the mistress of the house. He said he was kinda nervous to click the "read" button, as he couldn't be 100 percent sure, despite signs, that all had gone well with a threesome scene of razor's-edge edge play. But, WTH. Click. Read. Whoaaa, she was asking to . . . do it all over again, *and* with more ante-ing up. When I asked Mr. H what happened the second time around, he flashed a Cheshire cat smirk and glanced up, avoiding eye contact, rubbed his goateed chin, and, in a mocking James Bond tone, said, "That's for the next book." He won't tell. *Sad face.* Maybe too much wildness for a kiss 'n' tell? Okay, I submit. *Merci.* Game over.

The Switch: "You're the Boss, Applesauce!"[2]

The sexy-smarty sex therapist Venus Nicolino—Dr. V to those hooked on *LA Shrinks* (Bravo TV)—recently appeared on Andy Cohen's show, *Watch What Happens Live.* During a segment on guilty pleasures, she was asked, "What's the one thing women should try, sexually?" She blurted out what everyone expected to hear: "Anal!" Then she laughed, took it back, and said, "No, I would say try being sexually domineering in bed." She said that her clients who have tried it love it! Woohooo, well all right! Ride 'em, sexy cowgirls. Brav-A!

Even though it doesn't qualify as extreme play, the scenario in which the woman plays the role of the dominant appears in this section because it's uncommon (outside the dungeon) and considered way more "kinky" to the public. After all, scenes with a woman playing dominatrix are chosen by TV scriptwriters to add shock value. (And what does that say to us?!)

The cookie-cutter psychological profile of a professional roleplaying dom or domme presents a man or woman who kicks ass in life or career and is dominant by nature. The flipside corollary is that such domineering individuals often like to play submissive roles sexually (in the dungeon and at home), just as those with more submissive, less aggressive personalities may enjoy taking control in the bedroom. I've found much supporting evidence for the thesis and find it credible.

Let's say you are partnered with a hard-charging man whose perfect 10 on the psychological assessment chart fairly screams ALPHA MALE. He's domineering on the home front as well as in the workplace. No one anyone wants to tangle with. He's a restless sort, maybe has a wandering eye, seems a bit bored in bed. Wellll, this is going to sound counterintuitive, but I've seen enough, hanging around the scene, to know that you likely have a candidate for a switch routine. Surprised? I bet, but I submit herewith an axiom derived from the dungeon wisdom of the all-knowing *(believe it!)* dommes:

Betas see shrinks. Alphas visit dommes.

Trust those mistresses of the night, who have as much cause to celebrate a bonanza year on Wall Street as the city's Maserati dealer (in this, trust *me*!). Your strong-arming businessman-bully-by-day longs for release from captivity no less than his time clock–punching minions. All are work slaves, they to him and he to his driving striving. But whereas his frustrated underlings can go home and act out their stifled delusions of grandeur in lording it over the wife and the cocker spaniel, he's already King of the Hill, with nowhere to go but . . . down. Yes, he may surprise even himself to discover what relief and pleasure can ripple from the simple act of unfurling an iron fist. Ceding control to another, being treated as he's never treated in life, becoming a follower, a yes man: These are new experiences for the autocrat, who soon comes to see what stressful burdens he shoulders as Commander-in-Chief. And the experience of role-playing the submissive is transformative, as I've seen for myself and as you may behold, as well. Relieved of the crushing weight, your "new man" can find it hot to take commands from his lovemaking partner. He may be the boss of the house (this isn't likely to change, unless you come to savor the assertive role—bet you will!—and progressively begin to act on it), but in bed he will find he's secretly intrigued and excited to be toppled from his perch. In fact, most men tell me that they find it sexually arousing (on occasion) to be the "taker" in bed. They also appreciate how charged up the commanding role seems to make the female partner—"oozing lust like a sex-crazed nymph," in the poetic words of one fellow.

So let's try turning the DSRP tables. Now, while I do think most men like a light taste of their own medicine, I don't suggest just up and grabbing your guy, slapping a dog collar on him, and spanking him till he howls like some gimpy wimp. For the newbie, it's better to start things off using no props, just physical actions such as pinning down his hands, maybe a bit of biting, nipple squeezing, and hair pulling. If the fervor unleashed by acting the dominant then leads you to "ravage" your man, the thrill of your where-did-*that*-come-from? action as well as his impassioned reaction may surprise you both. *Thrillingly* and memorably.

In my pro domming days, my client list ranged from shy, meek men to cocksure SOBs and included rich, risk-taking men with gambling addictions, tough bikers, actors, car mechanics, CEOs, doctors, and others in positions of power. And I'd estimate that more than 90 percent of these male submissives told me that their wives had no idea they saw dominatrices and had no suspicion that they liked to be dominated in role play. When I asked if they could see their wives playing the dominant, many said yes but said they feared being left if they divulged their kinky fantasies. Some brave boys (admittedly, most were Europeans) said that they had confessed their predilections and were surprised at how accepting their wives had been. They had initiated dom/sub switch play within their relationships but still enjoyed the occasional "night out" with a pro domme. (Surprisingly—or not?—I know many pro dommes who have married their sub male clients, and I hear that those marriages are going strong.) What I'm hinting at is that you may make a *huuuge* discovery—one that could jazz up and strengthen your marriage or relationship.

Though I'm not into sexually dominating my lovers and Mr. H is not into being sexually submissive, he once did express an interest in and attraction to being ravaged by a woman. It happened recently, during the period when I was writing this book. We were lying in bed, I watching *Girls* on HBO and he reading Edgar Allan Poe on his iPhone—as you see, a thoroughly modern couple. I had watched Lena Dunham in season one episodes get DSRP-dommed by a struggling actor-type boy, in full-on BDSM style, sans toys. Watching this second-season show, I saw Lena do a full 180. On the streets of Brooklyn, she struck up a conversation with a rich doctor and jumped at his invitation to come home with him. Once inside the house, back to the floor, legs in air, she turned the tables and pushed the guy onto his back on the floor, climbed on top of him, and, through aggressive body language, made it clear that she was taking charge.

Rather stunned at the turn of events, I asked Mr. H if he thought he might like being dominated sexually by a woman. Like "don't move, don't speak" *commanded.* He said, "Yeah, that can be very hot. Men as well as women like to be sexually teased in that way, even with mild face slapping." Whoooaa . . . *what?* This was my own I'll-be-darned moment, as I'd had not a clue that Mr. H could be into being even mildly dominated. Emboldened, I asked Mr. H if, in fact, he'd ever had a woman completely sexually dominate him. He first said, "Uhhh . . . not really," then, "Wait, yeah, one time."

The story is, he'd met a cute, slightly built girl wearing a bubble-gum ponytail and Girl Scout–style khaki shorts at a bar. She was from Central America and said she was an activist in her country's freedom movement. He took her home and, like, as soon as they hit the bedroom, she *rahhhhhhhh!* ripped her hair free from the ponytail band and blind-sided him with a Judo-esque drop to the floor. He was like, "Holy shit . . . WTF!" I said, "Ha, was she, like, 'raping' you?" He said, "Yeah, kinda." I asked if it was hot. "It was. It made me go after her even more in returning her sexual dominant moves." So it was a brief switch, not a full-on dominatrix role play, and she told him that she liked being dommed by him as well.

See? You just don't know unless you ask. Without going to extremes, you can be the sexual dominant in role play, switching back and forth as the mood strikes. You might even start by dismissively rolling your eyes and engaging in playful verbal humiliation while you yourself are the sub, tied up, perhaps, and being spanked. The trick in being his dominant is to play things salty/sweet. Too much salt might turn him off, so give him a treat, sexually, after a stiff rebuke, command, or pain pinch. You might discover in reading his reactions that he *does* want you to "be the boss, Applesauce" . . . all the way home. Hey, hey! You might like it, too!

Switching back and forth—pinning him down before he whips you around to pin you—sounds like a virtual back-and-forth whirlwind of visceral, beasty sex—not a bad turn of events. Hmmm. Now, I've yet to try the sexual she-domme thing with my lover but I feel I could be tempted to give it a try . . .

On second thought, I think I'll stick with what works for me: alpha chick in public, letting loose by submitting in bed. And you?

LET'S NOW TALK ABOUT ENDING A kink relationship, whether you've been a light weekend player or a round-the-clock lifestyle partner. From the home front, I share some on-topic, breaking news: Mr. H and I remain best friends but are no longer a couple. After seven years, we began to realize that our ambitions for the future were no longer convergent. (No, *not* the "itch" thing, the sexual attraction's still there . . . anyway, I refuse to be a statistic.) We parted amicably, and I did the parting. Lucky for me, Mr. H is a stand-up good guy and now my dear friend and has dutifully erased all the kinky "compromising" pictures he took of me during play to add to our scenes. In retrospect, I consider that I was naive and reckless in allowing him to take them. What if he'd felt scorned and become vengeful? He might now be holding me hostage with racy bondage shots. So, vow to self and advice to readers: Don't ever let your partner take "incriminating" pictures or video of you unless it is on your own equipment—cell phone, camera, or video cam. No matter how hot it seems at the time to let a partner shoot and secret away blackmail-worthy scene pix or vids of you, it's just plain *stupid* and never worth the risk. Further, it's an even wiser idea to ban cameras altogether during play. I say this because, in the spirit of play, many kinksters find it a fun idea to "shoot their scenes." Think about it: Is one ever sure what the camera is catching? Even with no compromising sexual images, will you be cool with "coming out" to the world via images that unmistakably disclose "racy romp"? How to explain? On that same cautionary note, if you attend a kink party, you might choose to wear a fanciful Venetian costume mask, if you're determined to keep your private kink whims private.

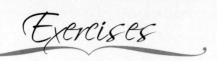

Exercises

*These final exercises are passive. Use them to find inspiration
in the alluring expression of eroticism as high art, where the idea
of taboo is continually up for revision.*

1. *Visit a supremely gifted photographer's portfolio on the web (www.
leb-photography.com).*

I once did a photo shoot for an exquisite collection of erotic S&M-themed photographs at the invitation of the boldly creative photographer Laurent E. Badessi.[3] Badessi asked that I write a brief sentence or two on BDSM for his personal dossier of the models' feelings about S&M. I wrote, "S&M is a natural dance between the dominant and the submissive dancers." He loved that. I love him. I was born to dance to his tunes. Badessi's works are part of the permanent collection of Le Musée des Arts Décoratifs at the Louvre in Paris. Go to Google Images to see Badessi's enkindling work. And while you're at it, you might check out the erotically charged black and white photographs of Robert Mapplethorpe and Helmut Newton, once banned by mainstream institutions and publications, now revered by same.

2. *Watch (grainy black and white but early, rare) footage of the breathtaking
Isadora Duncan (www.youtube.com/watch?v=mKtQWU2ifOs).*

I remember being taken as a very young child to see an exhibition on fashion and costumes of the early 1920s at the Metropolitan Museum of Art. I was blown away, frozen, rendered wide-eyed and rapt, by a tableau of mannequins in costumes that were thrilling and unlike any of the other droll 1920s outfits. These were long flowing dresses, draped with elaborate trailing scarves in a flamboyant display of artistic expression. I pointed at the foremost mannequin and demanded to know, *"Who is that!?"* and my mother said, "That's Isadora Duncan. She was a famous modern dancer who performed barefoot." She rented the

1968 Redgrave film for me, and for years thereafter I dressed up as the fascinating Isadora, pairing crazy long scarves with diaphanous Indian print tunics (there are still Polaroids around, ugh). I danced around the living room, flying off the couch and leaping onto the coffee table. In nursery school, I painted wildly bombastic watercolors. Stunned teachers declared, "This child will be an artist!" (My artist father said, "Break her fingers.") Might it be said that I was born with Duncan's spirit of abandon, which she awakened in me as she did in her followers? I think so. In her time, this freedom fighter for naturalistic, go-with-the-flow dance was considered eccentric and wanton, and she was banned from many venues for her wild expression of creativity—her "kink," as her detractors surely saw it, and as I here choose to call it, approvingly.

3. *Thrill to two greatest hits in one: an ice-dancing routine and a classic of twentieth-century music.*

Google the YouTube video of Jayne Torvill and Christopher Dean's 1984 Olympic couples' ice dancing routine, performed to the stirring score of Ravel's *Boléro*. It's said to be the most magical, beautiful, and sensational couple's dance in Olympic and even ice dance history. The two skaters blend as one, exuding overt sensual attraction even as each vies for dominance. At the end, he thrashes her body violently into the air and then flings her across the ice as he falls gracefully in line with her body. Perfect 6.0s across the board from the judges! Viewing the performance now, from a newly cultivated perspective, I recognize subtle S&M top and bottom moves and a physically harsh S&M-y role-playing finale. Passion incarnate, I call it, and offer it up as the paragon of everything awakening, inflaming, and wonderful that your DSRP can be.

THUS, I CONCLUDE THIS *POSH GIRL'S Guide to Play* in celebration of the voluptuous expression of beauty and ecstasy. That is what draws me into the dark, seductive passages of DSRP. The underlying tension of sensual warfare, the sense that at any moment the erotic tease, the dance, will erupt in operatic brutality, is the most erotic feeling imaginable. And the ability to communicate this unrestrained rapture through the visual and performing arts is the great achievement of the artists I here extol. It is not enough to read about DSRP. You must *see and experience* it for yourselves.

ISADORA DUNCAN ONCE WROTE,
"You were once wild here. Don't let them tame you."[4]

Oh, Isadora . . . Yes! Yes! Harder! Yes!

FINIS!

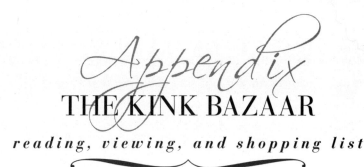

Appendix
THE KINK BAZAAR
reading, viewing, and shopping list

Herewith, the Posh Girl's Guide to all things koolly kink. *Kinky* sounds like *quirky*, in my book, so our shopping list of erotic books and films runs—*quirkily!* The recommended fiction ranges from *de rigueur novels* (because they're steamy classics, you understand—not because we have to) to unsung or forgotten works to books hot off the hard drive. Sex-themed nonfiction. American, Asian, and European films. Online adult sites. Kink provisions (where to buy). And finally, my advice on where to go kink-partner hunting, online and off, in your own back-yard and def off the beaten (ahem) trail. We all know there are jackals out there—they may look and act like trusty doggies but they're mean little critters, known to attack small and weakened prey—so it might be smart when hunting to ask a slew of questions before pouncing.

Posh Book List

FIFTY SHADES OF GREY by E. L. James. But of course. Or just wait for the movie.

JUSTINE by Marquis de Sade. The book that sent him to prison. The translation by Austryn Wainhouse (Grove Press) is the only complete American edition.

KAMA SUTRA. Ahhh, the Bible. Anyone into sex should read this informative book.

LOVERS' MASSAGE: SOOTHING TOUCH FOR TWO by Darrin Zeer. Ramp up that bondage massage.

VENUS IN FURS by Leopold von Sacher-Masoch. A classic, first published in Austria in 1870. Sexy, funny. A play based on the book premiered off-Broadway in 2010 (it was *something*, and female star Nina Arianda *sizzled*!), and Roman Polanski unveiled his film version, *Venus in Fur* [sic], starring his wife, Emmanuelle Seigner, at the Cannes Film Festival in May 2013.

STORY OF O by Pauline Réage (pseudonym of Anne Desclos). Now a classic, first published in 1954. Scenes of bondage, demonic desire, whips, masks, and chains, so explicit that early readers were convinced it was written by a man. Author Graham Greene wrote: "A rare thing, a pornographic book well written and without a trace of obscenity."

THE HAPPY HOOKER by Xaviera Hollander. Feisty memoir from the Dutch madame, detailing her bondage and fetish services.

TWO KNOTTY BOYS BACK ON THE ROPES by Two Knotty Boys. For those who want to spend more time on complex bondage techniques, here are 750 pages of photographs showing rope-tie positions. (This is their sequel to *Showing You the Ropes*.)

MY SECRET GARDEN: WOMEN'S SEXUAL FANTASIES. Women confide their sexual dreams. *My Mother/My Self: The Daughter's Search for Identity*. Why we become our mothers (in ways that may not suit). Both by Nancy Friday.

THE HITE REPORT: A NATIONWIDE STUDY OF FEMALE SEXUALITY by Shere Hite. Helped fuel the sexual revolution by explaining us to us.

HOW TO THINK MORE ABOUT SEX (THE SCHOOL OF LIFE) by Alain de Botton. Covers lust, fetishism, adultery, and pornography . . .

everything but vanilla, because maybe there is no vanilla?? Botton writes in his intro, "Few of us are remotely normal sexually." Hmmmm.

The Sleeping Beauty Trilogy by Anne Rice. Yes, she of the vampire novels. She wrote this one under a pseudonym in 1983, and it was reissued under more favorable social conditions in 2012. Why did she write it? "I decided to write the pornography I wanted to read, to prove that good S&M porn could be done without murder, burning, cutting or any kind of real physical harm; that a delicious pornography of detailed S&M games—dominance and submission, humiliation and love—could be made, all of it with elegance, refinement, and some romance." Read the entire interview at http://www.examiner.com/article/anne-rice-talks-about-the-sleeping-beauty-trilogy-fifty-shades-and-porn.

Or you could just slide your mouse over to good ol' free Wikipedia. I just discovered they have a huge section of photos on various bondage positions, including "head bondage"—WTH is that? http://en.wikipedia.org/wiki/List_of_bondage_positions. *C'est wow!*

Posh Kink-Themed Movies

Secretary. A must. Just when you're ready to give up on doormat Lee, played by Maggie Gyllenhaal, she pulls out some tricks of her own.

9 ½ Weeks. Another must. Just how far can things go? Mickey Rourke shows us.

The Lover. Based on the exquisite novel by Marguerite Duras, drawing from her own experience in girlhood.

Claire's Knee. (1971) French film starring Claire's knee as fetish object . . . an interesting one.

Caligula. Of coooourse . . . kink-o-rama.

IN THE REALM OF THE SENSES. Japanese film from the seventies. A sensual must . . . but very racy and extreme. Be warned.

QUILLS. Starring Kate Winslet and Geoffrey Rush. The last days of the indomitable Marquis De Sade, now an inmate in a Napoleonic-era insane asylum, where he fights a battle of wills against a tyrannical and prudish doctor.

THREE DAYS OF THE CONDOR. (1975) A must-see starring a hot young Robert Redford and a sultry Faye Dunaway. In a powerful DRSP-esque scene, Redford (a good guy but a desperado here) holds Dunaway captive (at gunpoint, on her bed), and the heat melts the screen. They begin a romance.

EMMANUELLE. The classic erotic movie of modern cinema, from 1974 . . . S&M-y.

THE DAMNED and *THE NIGHT PORTER*. Worlds apart from the tame-by-contrast workplace shenanigans of *Secretary*, these two films by Italian directors, both featuring Dirk Bogarde and Charlotte Rampling, are both rich with inspiration for scene setting and costuming. Luchino Visconti's *The Damned* (1969) lavishly, sensuously portrays the sadomasochism and transvestism rampant in Weimar Germany. Liliana Cavani's notorious *The Night Porter* (1974) memorably (and *controversially*) dramatizes Nazi sadomasochism. The iconic scene of Rampling performing a Marlene Dietrich song for lustful Nazi officers may be taste enough. Check it out on the web: www.youtube.com/watch?v=RUz RoSwPLRA.

CINEKINK. A high-end kink film festival. You can check out their audience choice awards on their website (http://cinekink.com). Their films can be purchased at http://astore.amazon.com/cine0f-20.

Posh DSRP Websites

For all things kink posh, I invite you to visit the *The Posh Girl's Guide to Play* website. Bloggie treats, tips, Q&A, and callouts for hot new stuff to do, read, watch, and buy. And to come, vlogs and sexy videos. littleblackhandcuffs.com.

BDSM Adult Film Sites Featuring Sub Girls in Adult XXX-Rated Very Racy Films (Posh? Uhhh, Not So Much)

These sites, which feature sub girls in XXX-rated (very, very, very racy) films, offer extreme fare, but they can spark your imagination and might be fun to watch with a lover, as long as he's someone you can trust not to get the "wrong ideas."

RESTRAINED ELEGANCE (www.restrainedelegance.com). Racy, fun, and, yes, kinda porno-y sleazy, but one of the best of the triple-X girl-porn video sites, with free pix and vid trailers. They seem to be marketing more toward men, as in some scenes they will feature a female boss and female secretary. Oo la la. But! You might take inspiration from the costumes and plots, and you may see a bondage position you like. The women are beautiful, BTW, and the production is very tastefully mastered, for XXX-rated fare.

AASIA'S BONDAGE (www.aasiasbondage.com). This site has free sub girl/male dom stories, rated by readers, and free racy sub girl play photos. It also has a fine selection of adult sub girl/male dom clips—the porno version of *Fifty Shades*. Might be fun to watch some X-rated bondage in private or with your lover. Again, good for stoking the imagination and giving you some *fresh* ideas. *Wink*.

GOOGLE. There's always the Google approach to accessing free soft-core bondage videos or photos, where you'll find the less sleazy of the sleaze. You can pick and choose which videos you want to watch based on cover photos. Some will be more artistic and "polite" than others.

The Posh Kink Cache
(A Collection of Hidden and Forbidden Treasures)

The lingerie is scrumptious, the costume selection eclectic, and the toys first-rate and plentiful. Let's start with the finery and costumes.

AGENT PROVOCATEUR (www.agentprovocateur.com). Upscale lingerie store catering to kinksters and frequented by movie stars, with movie-star prices to match. Sometimes they have great sales, and I must say their stuff is beautifully designed and constructed, worth the price and the occasional splurge. Also, they have high-end fun kink toys like rhinestone headed crops and glam blindfolds.

KIKI DE MONTPARNASSE (www.kikidm.com). Great lingerie but even better kink toys, from silk bow handcuffs and French lace blindfolds to gold-plated mini vibrators, twenty-four-carat gold handcuffs, and exotic faux alligator paddles and floggers. Ooo la la.

FRÄULEIN KINK (www.frauleinkink.com). Great lingerie that's top-of-the-line, sophisticated kink, and splendid kink toys: fur handcuffs and 1920s-style flapper fringe blindfolds.

RICKY'S (www.rickysnyc.com). New York City women luvvvv Ricky's. It's where they indulge their caprices for unique fashion items and costumes, naughty novelties, makeup and hair products, introductory "sex and mischief" kits. Talk about quirky! Maybe all you need to hear is that Ricky's is also a fave with transvestites, so you absolutely know that everything in the store is going to be fab-o-licious! Stores all over town, as you'll see on the site.

DARKESTAR (www.darkestar.com) Their motto is "Get tied up in fashion," and chic Vogue-ish cuffs and couture and a posh bondage bed pillow with built-in silk hand ties and blindfold should do it!

Posh Kink Toy Sites

For you, this will be like taking your kid-self to a toy store. Grab what you like and you'll instantly figure out how to play with it, though, of course, there's no one "correct" way. Yes, there are some electrical devices that will require reading the manual, and there are lots of "hitting" toys (avoid the kidney area). That's 'bout as complicated as it gets.

STOCKROOM (www.stockroom.com). An upscale (not cheap and sleazy) site for toys, but the prices are low to medium range. It's a kink candy store of sexy toys, fun bondage restraints, and even kink furniture. Check it out just for kicks at least!

FETISHTOYBOX (www.fetishtoybox.com). This is where you can find all the toys we have discussed. Nice selection of the best kink how-to books, to dig in deeper. From Pyrex dildos to more advanced toys like electric dildos that you attach to a gizmo with knobs to heighten the pulses or temps, from pleasurable low pulses to more shock-y ones. Also, toys such as electric straps you can comfortably place on your private parts, while your partner holds a small/discreet control pad to send you a teeny shock, under the five-star restaurant table, perhaps. Oo la la la la. Just click around the site, choose entry-level toys, and give yourself a few months of play activity and party conversation with some cool, like-minded people to branch out to kinkier choices to fill your toy box. Or not.

QUALITY WHIPS BY VICTOR TELLA (www.snakewhip.com) and MURPHY WHIPS (www.murphywhips.com). If you want to explore, you might want to give a whip a go. Atomic bomb red flag warning though. That said, Snakewhip.com is quality but the less expensive option, while Aussie Michael Murphy is the best in the business. A nice as hell guy, too. (Note: The wait time for custom-made whips will be months but worth it. They feel like animal spirit incarnate (truly)— smooth, flexible as a real snake body, and next level. Even the submissive might want to crack the whip just for fun.) Start with a single-tail whip, which startles with an exciting crack noise for instant submissive psychological shock *without* even touching the body. If wielded correctly, however, this device can gently deliver the submissive a little tiny sting on the arse. WARNING: One needs lots of practice with single-tails before engaging in play. Professional dommes say that one should be expert enough—as *they* are, I can testify—to be able to flip a light switch on and off with a crack of the whip before even *thinking about* landing a hit on a player. Should be damn close, anyway! After achieving some degree of mastery, try putting out a candle flame. It's extremely empowering to feel like Sheena, Queen of the Jungle, gripping and cracking the lash used to tame the kings of the jungle, and maybe your "king"?? (Note: Those who passed on the previous Taboo chapter may want to check out the brief switching section therein.) I've pulled out the single-tail whip at many a house party and grinned (well, more like smirked) watching all the vanilla-world people having a whip-cracking good time. Mostly they chose to whip a wall, but sometimes they aimed at each other, lightly and in the spirit of play. Hmmmm, men and women breaking out. As I wrote in chapter 12, BTW, most single-tail whips are sold for use in whip-cracking contests at Wild West shows, not for the practice of BDSM. Note: I do not condone whipping or any other strikes to the body, unless it's done very gently, intending and causing no harm.

Posh Kink-Partner Hunting

If you are looking for a partner who's not so much kink-obsessed as up for dabbling, then I suggest *not* going to a kink dating site but to a vanilla one, and simply hinting that you are interested in, and maybe interested in trying, some DSRP or light BDSM. Or that you might be interested in exploring some kink—with the right person. Mr. H has met most of his kink girl partners through OkCupid. None of these women were experienced with DSRP but wanted to talk about it and maybe try it. Communicating through a neutral dating site will cut the chances of your conversing with an experienced 24/7 male dom who might be waaay too kinky or kink-obsessed for you.

OKCUPID.COM. It's free, it's hip, and more Facebook-y than other sites, and you won't be out of place hinting at your kinky interests. Hell, these days, you can bring up light kink even on Christian dating sites. It's not a strict taboo anymore, if you recall my report in chapter 4, where I discussed digging around some religious dating message boards and finding slews of people eager to try BDSM.

FETLIFE.COM. For a more sophisticated kink crowd than you'll find on the average kink site. This is the "cool kid" Facebook of kink, with users ranging from billionaires (yes, 'tis true; I know a very nice one who has a FetLife profile) to solid career men and women to awesome artists. In addition to social networking, they also have a great selection of high-end kink store and kink services ads, including one for a legal service, the first I've seen, for women who are into submissive DSRP. I would stay away from the other popular and large kink community sites. I won't call them out, but the fare, predominantly, is sleaze-ridden and intentionally degrading to women.

Kink Parties

FETLIFE is also a good place to find kink parties in your area. In my experience, the huge majority of party guests are well educated and well off, "normal" people who get together in order to party where everyone is simply okay with kink. Most are not freaky-deaky kinky orgies. Great way to meet a partner or share an evening with other free-minded people. At one such party, a good friend met an emergency room surgeon who practices in Manhattan, and off they went to a great relationship, dabbling in some kink, on and off. Planning a trip across the pond one day soon? I saw a FetLife ad for a kink store in London where sub girls can pay to get spanked or otherwise play out their kinky desires (www.londonsubmissivegirls.com). To find parties on FetLife, get yourself a free profile and click on the "event" section.

SANCTUM CLUB (www.sanctumclub.com). Big news out of Los Angeles: In March 2013 came whispers of this new *Eyes Wide Shut* fetish nightclub—exclusive, clandestine, expensive. Membership is $2,000 to $4,500 (for the level V room); guest admittance is $250. Members and guests, ladies and gents, admitted by approval only. Hey, maybe you'll run into Prince Harry in a Venetian Diablo mask?! Seriously, would *not* surprise moi, to judge from my experience attending secrète, très expensive fetish parties. Mum's the word! The founders (posh characters, both with art-world cred) say they're putting "eroticism front and center, with a mix of theater and fetish culture," and *LA Times* reporter August Brown describes the club as having "an aesthetic that's half pagan sex cult, half entertainment-mogul after-party." He quotes the male partner as saying, "We want people to take sensuality seriously," and that his concept for Sanctum was "a mix of Illuminati imagery . . . and bondage erotica, all given a gentlemanly veneer . . . [an] effort to incorporate underground fetish culture into exclusive bottle-service terrain." And from the female partner: "I'm also a biologist with a real strong interest in animal and insect sexuality . . . I still have no idea how humans evolved to have the most vanilla sexuality of any species." "L.A.'s Gulfstream set has never needed prodding to explore their lustful curiosity," Brown writes. "But Sanctum is a new, secretive place for them to try it on." He further quoted the male partner as saying, "I have no desire for a swingers' party here, but I do want to open up a dialogue about how we can come out of our fear of sexuality." To which I can hear Posh Girls everywhere responding, "What took you so long?!" Sounds amazing! No?

And in Special, Hearty Tribute . . .

I would like to give a *huuuge* posh-shout-out to a wonderful, singularly dedicated, proactive, and hands-on organization that fights tirelessly "for sexual freedom and privacy rights for all adults who engage in safe, sane, and consensual behavior" (taken from the "About Us" section of their website): the National Coalition for Sexual Freedom. The coalition is headed by a noteworthy and *très, très* cool woman named Susan Wright. She really steps up to come to the rescue of individuals discriminated against because of their sexual preferences. Check out their site, and toss them a few bucks if you're feeling Posh Girl kinky benevolent humanitarian: www.ncsfreedom.org.

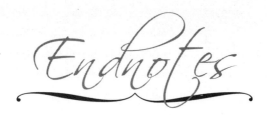

Endnotes

chapter one

1. Kayt Sukel. "50 Shades of Grey (Matter): How Science Is Defying BDSM Stereotypes." *Huffington Post*, May 30, 2012.

2. We will address your "un-like" list and your erotic story or stories later, so keep these tucked away in your private email or handwrite them by candlelight, eighteenth-century maiden's chamber style, and then fold them up and stash them in your lingerie drawer. Do make a lingerie drawer, as you will be buying new lingerie for your exciting role-play-theater encounters with your lover.

chapter two

1. A good choice, from an unknockable source: Matt Haber. "A Hush-Hush Topic No More." *The New York Times*, February 27, 2013.

chapter three

1. Rachel R. White. "The Story of 'No': S&M Sex Clubs Sprout Up on Ivy Campuses, and Coercion Becomes an Issue." *The New York Observer*, November 16, 2012.

chapter four

1. Dana Goldstein. "On Feminism and Sadomasochistic Sex." *The Nation* (blog), April 16, 2012.

2. E. Hariton. "Women's Fantasies During Sexual Intercourse with their Husbands: A Normative Study with Tests of Personality and Theoretical Models." Unpublished doctoral dissertation, City University of New York. 1970.

3. Camille Paglia. "Scholars in Bondage." *The Chronicle of Higher Education*, May 20 2013. http://chronicle.com/article/Scholars-in-Bondage/139251/.

4. T. K. V. Desikachar with R. H. Cravens. *Health, Healing, and Beyond: Yoga and the Living Tradition of T. Krishnamacharya*. New York: North Point Press, 1998.

5. Ibid.

6. Fernando Pagés Ruiz. "Krishnamacharya's Legacy." *Yoga Journal*, May/June 2001. http://www.yogajournal.com/wisdom/465?page=2

7. Phil Catalfo. "Is Yoga a Religion?" *Yoga Journal*. http://www.yogajournal.com/lifestyle/283.

8. T. K. V. Desikachar. *The Heart of Yoga: Developing a Personal Practice*. Rochester, VT: Inner Traditions, 1999.

9. Desikachar with Cravens. *Health, Healing, and Beyond*.

10. Ibid.

11. Desikachar. *The Heart of Yoga*.

chapter five

1. The 2001 MTV Video Music Awards aired live on September 6, 2001, honoring the best music videos from June 10, 2000, to June 8, 2001. The show was hosted by Jamie Foxx at the Metropolitan Opera House in New York City.

2. "Sweaty T-Shirts and Human Mate Choice." http://www.pbs.org/wgbh/evolution/library/01/6/l_016_08.html.

chapter seven

1. Aljean Harmetz. *The Making of Casablanca: Bogart, Bergman, and World War II*. New York: Hyperion, 2002, 169.

2. "Jill Krementz Covers Duane Michals." *New York Social Diary*, March 6, 2013.

chapter eight

1. Sarah Baring (obituary). *Telegraph*. February 15, 2013.
2. Nate C. Hindman. The Huffington Post, February 21, 2013. http://www.huffingtonpost.com/2013/02/21/taxitreats-condom-vending-machines_n_2735647.html
3. Live and learn. Even in New York City, I've discovered, it's possible to stock an enviable DSRP wardrobe closet at budget prices. In every neighborhood of Manhattan, there are resale and vintage shops selling fabulous castoffs at every price point. And for shopping really on the cheap, for all variety of costumes, I hit the charity chain shops, even rummage sales in the basements of Upper East Side churches with rosters of posh and generous worshippers. Contact me on littleblackhandcuffs.com and I'll send you my insider list!

chapter nine

1. And besides, I love insinuating a guy with Burton's renegade rep into these pages. As Elizabeth Weitzman wrote in the *New York Daily News*, "Burton rarely worries about what can or should be done; he just goes ahead and does it." Like!
2. Alan Riding. "Arts Abroad; Picasso's Carnal Carnival." *The New York Times*, March 22, 2001.
3. Sukel, "50 Shades of Grey (Matter)."
4. Gwen Lawrence. "Pose of the Month: Bow Pose." Active.com. http://beta.active.com/yoga/articles/pose-of-the-month-bow-pose.

chapter twelve

1. Jillian Keenan. "We're Kinky, Not Crazy." *Slate*, March 8, 2013.
2. Borrowing starstruck Andy Warhol's famous words to muse Edie Sedgwick (*Factory Girl*, 2006)
3. One of the images (not mine) appeared as a thirty-by-sixty-foot billboard above Times Square for a Charles Jourdan ad campaign.
4. Isadora Duncan. *Isadora Speaks: Writings & Speeches of Isadora Duncan*. Chicago: Charles H Kerr, 1994.

appendix

1. Nola Cancel. "Anne Rice Talks About the 'Sleeping Beauty' Trilogy, 'Fifty Shades' and Porn." Examiner.com, June 11, 2012.

2. August Brown, "Sanctum Duo Aim to Give L.A. a Fresh Dose of Sexuality," *Los Angeles Times*, March 29, 2013..

Acknowledgments

The synchronicity of the *K*'s. Thank you to my best friend and mother, Karen; my lit guru, Katie; my deceased childhood soul mate, Kat; my college confederate in roguery, Katie; my heroine agent, M. Kaffel; and my championing editor, Laura K. Mazer. When I was twelve, a psychic at a Spence School classmate's Harvard Club bat mitzvah party told me that women, not men, would help me in life and that he saw the letter *K*. To all the femme *K*'s, you are my wickedly brilliant angels.

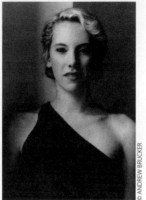

© ANDREW BRUCKER

About the Author

Alexis Lass's well-rounded education took place at the Spence School, the Kent School, Bard College, University of Bologna, and the American Academy of Dramatic Arts. She worked as a Certified Yoga Instructor and did some stage and television work in New York City before taking on a brief stint as a pro Dominatrix.

For five years, Lass owned and operated her own fetish film production company in Manhattan. Her film *Infernali* won Best Picture Award at the Traum Film Festival in Germany, and the trailer was in the winner's circle for the best horror film trailer at the Paranoia Film Festival in Los Angeles.

In partnership with *Penthouse Magazine*, Lass ran fetish parties at Chris Noth's Cutting Room lounge in Manhattan, earning a Page Six spread of party pics in the New York *Post* as well as live video coverage on its website. She was featured in Katie Roiphe's essay collection *In Praise of Messy Lives*, and in a story by Roiphe on Slate.com.

Lass, who categorizes herself as "proper Bohemian," resides on the Upper East Side of Manhattan, is active with animal rights groups, and volunteers with a cat rescue group. You can learn more about her at littleblackhandcuffs.com.

Selected Titles from Seal Press

By women. For women.

Getting Off: A Woman's Guide to Masturbation, by Jamye Waxman, illustrations by Molly Crabapple. $15.95, 978-1-58005-219-1. Empowering and female-positive, this is a comprehensive guide for women on the history and mechanics of the oldest and most common sexual practice.

Dirty Girls: Erotica for Women, edited by Rachel Kramer Bussel. $15.95, 978-1-58005-251-1. A collection of tantalizing and steamy stories compiled by prolific erotica writer Rachel Kramer Bussel.

Mind-Blowing Sex: A Woman's Guide, by Diana Cage. $17.00, 978-1-58005-389-1. An instructive, accessible sexual guide that will help women and their partners make their sex life more empowering, exciting, and enjoyable.

Screw Everyone: Sleeping My Way to Monogamy, by Ophira Eisenberg. $16.00, 978-1-58005-439-3. Comedian Ophira Eisenberg's wisecracking account of how she spent most of her life saying "yes" to everything—and everyone—and how that attitude ultimately helped her overcome her phobia of commitment.

Yogalosophy: 28 Days to the Ultimate Mind-Body Makeover, by Mandy Ingber. $18.00, 978-1-58005-445-4. Celebrity yoga instructor Mandy Ingber offers a realistic, flexible, daily plan that will help readers transform their minds, their bodies, and their lives.

What You Really Really Want: The Smart Girl's Shame-Free Guide to Sex and Safety, by Jaclyn Friedman. $17.00, 978-1-58005-344-0. An educational and interactive guide that gives young women the tools they need to decipher the modern world's confusing, hyper-sexualized landscape and define their own sexual identity.

FIND SEAL PRESS ONLINE
www.SealPress.com
www.Facebook.com/SealPress
Twitter: @SealPress